This book is dedicated to the people with epilepsy whom I have been privileged to know over the past twenty years, who have taught me so much and from whom I continue to learn.

Foreword

Epilepsy is, obviously, a medical condition and it is to medicine that most people turn in the face of seizures. Yet, epilepsy is also a condition that impacts hugely on people's lives in areas such as schooling, driving, employment, planning a family, travel, insurance, sports, ageing, other illnesses, choosing a place to live, and just about every other aspect of life that you can imagine.

One thing, however, is certain. Epilepsy is not a simple topic and it is not a simple illness. While people living with epilepsy no doubt want to find out all they can once they have been diagnosed, when they have just started taking anti-epileptic medication they are probably not going to feel quite up to reading medical journals and textbooks.

If you have ever tried to buy a straightforward book about epilepsy, one that tells you how you might manage to live with it, chances are you didn't have much success. Good books do crop up from time to time, but they are few and far between. Good internet sites are much the same – they seldom tell you who wrote what you are reading, they are often not updated regularly, and the reliability of the information can vary greatly from site to site.

Understanding Epilepsy is one of those good books that occasionally finds its way into the health sections of bookstores. It is a very aptly titled book, because not only is it written with an obvious depth of understanding and clear authority – Neil Buchanan is Professor Emeritus of Medicine at the University of Sydney – it is written so that you will be able to make immediate sense of this age-old illness, even if you've never read anything else about it.

Understanding Epilepsy is not just about epilepsy as a medical condition. It is a very practical book for people who have to live with epilepsy, who will have a heap of questions, and who want to make the most of their personal circumstances so that they can get on with their lives.

People living with epilepsy include those who have epilepsy as well as those who live with someone else's epilepsy – that of a child, a partner, a sibling, a friend or, increasingly, a parent. After reading this book, you will know it really is possible to live a life that is rich and fulfilling, vigorous and happy, despite epilepsy. If you have epilepsy, it will challenge you and help you move forward.

Drawing upon his vast experience with epilepsy over many years, Neil is passionate about improving the lives of those diagnosed with it and his commitment to the epilepsy community at large is further evidenced by his willingness to accept the many invitations he receives to speak at public meetings and seminars.

This relatively small book provides technical information in language that you can understand. It covers so much – from diagnosis and testing to medications and other treatments, from pseudo-epileptic seizures to the issues of stigma and self-esteem, from social responsibility and the law to the classification of various types of epilepsy – and while guiding us through all this it somehow opens us all up to more possibilities in our lives than we had before we started to read it.

Russell Pollard
NATIONAL EXECUTIVE OFFICER, EPILEPSY AUSTRALIA

Denise Chapman
SERVICES MANAGER, EPILEPSY AUSTRALIA, NEW SOUTH WALES

Contents

Acknowledgments

I would like to thank Amanda Buxton, Robin Brown, Catherine Clifford, Edith and Robert Gourley, Dr Paddy Grattan-Smith, Diana Hills, Claire Lisle, Dr John Lisyak, Diana Sawyer and Dr Graham Scambler for their useful comments on the manuscript. I am also indebted to Pamela Garske for typing the manuscript. The contribution by Russell Pollard and Denise Chapman of the foreword is much appreciated.

Finally, the author and publisher are grateful to the following for permission to reproduce copyright material: Butterworth-Heinemann Ltd for extract from *Epilepsies of Childhood* by Nial O'Donahue (London, 1985); Penguin Books for extract from *The Puzzles of Childhood* by Manning Clark (Melbourne, 1989); and University of NSW Press for extract from *Regaining Compassion for Humanity and Nature* by Charles Birch (Sydney, 1993).

Preface

This book is a revision of previous books I have written on epilepsy. There have been substantial advances in epilepsy treatment in the past ten to fifteen years, with the advent of a number of new medications which are now in day-to-day use, an increase in investigational facilities and the greater recognition of the value of epilepsy surgery. A deeper understanding of the genetics of epilepsy is perhaps one of the most exciting developments in the pipeline, although at present this is only of limited value to individual patients and families.

There are not too many new medications in development at the time of writing this book, so it is important to use what we have to the best of our ability. This includes ensuring that people with epilepsy are well informed about their condition, the medications they are taking and the social implications of having epilepsy. I hope that this book may assist people with epilepsy, the parents and carers of people with epilepsy, and teachers and school counsellors.

Prologue

Going Forward

Since the early 1980s there has been a progressive, world-wide increase in interest in epilepsy with the development of a subspeciality in medicine called 'epileptology'. This interest has resulted in the development of epilepsy centres, especially in Western countries. One of the main roles of the centres is the testing of people who have severe problems with their epilepsy with a view to trying new treatments, including epilepsy surgery. These detailed investigations, using new technologies such as MR1, SPECT and PET scanning, have provided a great deal of useful information about epilepsy in general, as well as allowing a number of people with uncontrollable epilepsy to be helped by epilepsy surgery.

Over the past fifteen years there has been almost a doubling of the number of anti-epileptic medications available in day-to-day medical practice. This has not resolved the problems of many people with epilepsy, but it has allowed a greater choice of medications, and certainly some of the newer drugs have kinder side effects profiles than their predecessors. The development of further medications has slowed down substantially and we are in a phase of consolidation: learning to optimise the use of existing medications, that is, to achieve the best possible seizure control with the least side effects.

These improvements should diminish the number of people in society suffering uncontrolled seizures, which in turn should assist in reducing the social consequences of epilepsy. Seizures are unpredictable and frequently occur without warning; they can also be frightening to onlookers. Therefore any reduction in the number of people having seizures will be good not only for the individual, but also in terms of the general public's view of epilepsy as a condition.

For reasons that are quite understandable, many people with epilepsy are unwilling to discuss their condition. As the situation improves it will become more and more important for them to stand up and be counted in society – to demonstrate that despite their epilepsy they lead normal, or largely normal, lives. This book will not imply that they should advertise the fact that they have epilepsy, but will suggest that being more open about it will lead to acceptance of their own condition and probably an increased acceptance by society. Don't wait for 'famous' people to declare their epilepsy: go out there and do it yourself!

Chapter 1

The Social Perspective

We all expect to be ill from time to time, usually with quite short-lived illnesses such as the common cold or flu. We accept such ailments as part of life. However, some people will develop more chronic, or long-term, illnesses, of which epilepsy is but one example. No one wishes to develop such illnesses, but people who do so need to realise and subsequently accept that these conditions are also part of life.

The diagnosis of epilepsy is often associated with a feeling of gloom, that 'the end of the world' is at hand. That this is not so may be very hard for people with epilepsy, or parents of newly diagnosed children, to appreciate at the time. Luckily, for most people there is a progressive acceptance of their epilepsy over time – they accept it as being part and parcel of themselves, in the same way that they might accept having red hair, blue eyes or being overweight, and so on. The issue of acceptance is most important and will be discussed in some detail in Chapter 14.

As with other chronic conditions, epilepsy comes in varying degrees of severity. Many people with epilepsy have no significant problems at all. For some 60–70 per cent the condition is mild and well controlled by medication, and many of these people will eventually come off medication and remain seizure-free for the rest of their lives. It is likely that they will feel little or no need to discuss their condition publicly. Other individuals who have frequent seizures or newly diagnosed epilepsy will be more visible in society, and will therefore need the most support.

Epilepsy is somewhat different from other chronic conditions because of its social impact. The very unpredictability of seizures, in terms of their timing, severity and the situations in which they may occur, can cause social difficulties. People with epilepsy can be functioning quite normally one minute and having a seizure the next. It is understandable that they often feel they have no control over their condition. Indeed, they may feel that they have no control over their lives. This sense of losing control can be exacerbated by the restrictions that seizures sometimes place on career and lifestyle. All these factors are compounded by the discrimination, or stigma, associated with epilepsy; although, as we will see later, this is more often perceived than real.

The issue of stigma leads to a couple of prickly issues that should be tackled early on in any discussion of epilepsy: whether those suffering from the condition are 'epileptics' or 'people with epilepsy', and whether or not epilepsy is a disease. It has been argued by epilepsy associations, with good intent, that the stigma applied to epilepsy would be lessened if the term 'epileptic' were not used. They say that people with epilepsy should be seen as people first, epileptics second – that they shouldn't be identified so closely with their condition. Having thought about this for over a decade, and discussed it with many people with epilepsy, who use the word 'epileptic' to describe themselves anyway, I feel that the associations' approach is counterproductive. People with asthma call themselves 'asthmatics', diabetes, 'diabetics', arthritis, 'arthritics', and so on. Why should people with epilepsy drop out of the mainstream and be something different, something special? This specialness will only serve to isolate them further from people with other chronic conditions from whose experience they might draw solace.

Epilepsy associations have also encouraged people to refer to epilepsy as a symptom rather than a disease. A symptom of what, we might ask? This unwillingness to call epilepsy a disease arises from the mistaken perception that a disease is 'catchable'. But people who have seizures recognise that there is something amiss – namely, that they have epilepsy – whether or not they call it a symptom, a condition or a disease. It is suggested that 'political correctness' in this regard is of no intrinsic value, and will have no effect on the way in which the condition is viewed, either by epileptics themselves or by the general public.

Epilepsy is a medical condition, which is like other long-term illnesses in that it occurs over a range of severities. However, there are important differences in terms of social implications. The plea throughout this book is always to consider social aspects, as well as medical ones, in the day-to-day management of individuals with epilepsy.

Chapter 2

What is Epilepsy?

Epilepsy is a condition that is characterised by recurrent seizures. A seizure is an aberrant movement, thought process or feeling, which is caused by an abnormal discharge of electrical activity from the brain.

A number of words are used to describe seizures, including 'turns', 'blackouts', 'fits' and 'convulsions'. These are all intended to have the same meaning, but the preferred terms are 'seizures', 'fits' and 'convulsions'. The others cause confusion, as they also refer to non-epileptic events.

Some seizures are obvious to onlookers in that they consist largely of body movement (convulsive seizures), while others are only apparent to the person with epilepsy as there is little or nothing outwardly visible (non-convulsive seizures). During a seizure a person will suffer either a loss of awareness or total loss of consciousness. Some people will experience what they regard as a 'warning' in the form of an aura (an odd physical sensation, or perhaps a feeling of fear) before a major convulsion, but most seizures are of sudden, unexpected onset. So there are many different seizure types, which are of variable severity, in terms of both their nature and frequency.

There are also different types of epilepsy. In childhood these are often grouped into syndromes; for example, the Lennox-Gastaut Syndrome (discussed in more detail in Chapter 5) is classified as such because it has a particular presentation at a particular age, and runs a predictable course over time. However, as we shall see, a person with a particular epilepsy syndrome may exhibit more than one type of seizure as part of that syndrome, with some people showing predominantly one, and others several, seizure types.

The general public, as well as many people with epilepsy, do not appreciate the distinction between types of seizures and types of epilepsy. They do not realise that there are many different seizure types, which come in different degrees of severity, and numerous forms of epilepsy, each with a particular presentation and outlook. There is a sort of mind-set that 'all epilepsy is the same'. It is important for people with epilepsy to have an understanding of the subject as a whole, as well as an understanding of their own epilepsy, so that they can educate the public at large about the condition.

In nearly 75 per cent of cases epilepsy begins before the age of twenty, and approximately 6 per cent of children will have a seizure at some time during their childhood. The majority of these seizures, however, are related to fever (febrile convulsions) and do not lead to the development of epilepsy. At the other end of the spectrum, more older people are having seizures and subsequently developing epilepsy. This increase is attributable to the progressive ageing of the population in most Western countries, and has social and medical implications that will be discussed later.

A single fit does not in itself constitute a diagnosis of epilepsy, which by definition implies *having recurrent seizures*, so treatment with anti-epileptic drugs (AEDs) would not usually be commenced after a single seizure. There may be exceptions to this general rule, depending on the nature of the seizure, its timing and any underlying problems in the patient. For example, if a single seizure occurs in an individual with underlying brain damage, it is known that the chance of recurrence is about 90 per cent. Therefore, logic would suggest the use of medication. On the other hand, in people without any demonstrable brain abnormalities, the recurrence rate is about 50–60 per cent over the first year after a single seizure. This implies that if all individuals were to go onto an AED after a single seizure, 40–50 per cent of them might be taking medication unnecessarily.

It is also important to mention that there are many conditions that may mimic, but are *not*, epilepsy. It is generally accepted that up to 20 per cent of people referred to specialist epilepsy centres do not have epilepsy. It is vital that the correct diagnosis be reached so as not to commit a person to years of unnecessary treatment with medication, let alone subject them to the social implications of the diagnosis. If it is difficult to be sure if someone has epilepsy, it may be wise to observe the person on no medication to see what happens. Epilepsy is a recurrent condition that will eventually declare itself, and treatment can then be commenced.

The conditions that fall into the category of 'non-epilepsy' include:

- *Syncopal (fainting) episodes.*
- *Breath-holding attacks in children.*
- *Abnormalities of heart rhythm.*
- *Vertigo.*
- *Narcolepsy (continual desire to sleep).*
- *Hypnogogic jerks (jumping legs).* These are very common and affect most of us from time to time as we are drifting off to sleep. Because they occur so frequently they can be regarded as 'normal'.

- *Tics and rituals.* These include twitching of the face and blinking.
- *Night terrors in young children.*
- *Overbreathing (hyperventilation).* This is usually associated with an acute anxiety (panic) attack and is seen most often in young women. The overbreathing alters the chemical balance of the blood and may cause some mild muscular twitching of the hands, and pins and needles of the hands and around the mouth. Overbreathing may be used by a doctor, especially when dealing with children, to try to bring on a seizure to confirm the diagnosis of certain types of epilepsy.
- *Hypoglycaemia (low blood sugar).* This is an uncommon cause of seizures, but should always be excluded.
- *Behavioural problems.* It is common for children with behavioural problems such as temper tantrums or rage attacks to be referred with a suggested diagnosis of temporal lobe epilepsy. While there is no doubt that behavioural abnormalities can occur in those with temporal lobe epilepsy, this is quite uncommon. The vast majority of children with behavioural problems have exactly that – they do not have epilepsy.
- *Pseudo-epileptic seizures.* This is an important topic and will be dealt with in more detail later. In essence, pseudo-epileptic seizures are episodes that look like seizures, but are not. They may occur in people with or without epilepsy. They are used subconsciously to achieve some end, which in the simplest terms might be described as attention.

As will become apparent later, there are tests available that will sort out many, but not all, diagnostic problems. As a general rule, *if in doubt about the diagnosis of epilepsy, wait until it declares itself before commencing medication.* Discuss the pros and cons with your doctor and, if you think it might be helpful, obtain a second opinion.

When confronted with a possible diagnosis of epilepsy, there is information that you should obtain so as to have some understanding of the problem. The following questions may provide a useful starting point:

- Is it definitely epilepsy?
- What kind of epilepsy?
- What is the cause?
- What tests will be useful?
- Is treatment necessary?
- If so, what treatment and what are the side effects?
- How long will treatment be for?
- When, and how, will treatment be stopped?
- What is my role, as the person with epilepsy, in my own management?
- Where can I get more advice if I need it?

Naturally, not all of these questions will be asked at any one time, but over some months. Hopefully, the following chapters will assist you in answering some of them.

Chapter 3

The Causes of Epilepsy and Seizure-provoking Factors

There are many causes of epilepsy, which vary with the age at which seizures begin and the nature of the seizures. There are also a number of provoking (trigger) factors that may induce seizures. These factors do not bring on epilepsy itself, but can make seizures more frequent in some people with established epilepsy.

This chapter will explain the causes of epilepsy in general terms, before looking at more specific causes of the condition. It will also discuss some of the provoking factors that may induce seizures in those with epilepsy.

GENERAL CAUSES OF EPILEPSY

It is convenient, if not scientifically correct, to explain epilepsy as being of two types: primary, or idiopathic, epilepsy; and secondary epilepsy. This classification is quite artificial, but it is helpful in understanding how seizures arise.

Primary Epilepsy

If it is not possible to define the exact cause of an individual's epilepsy, it is said to be primary epilepsy. There may be an abnormality in exactly the same place in the brain as in someone with secondary epilepsy, but today's tests do not reveal the abnormality. As the tests become more precise, the cause of epilepsy will be found in more and more individuals, so the number of people with primary epilepsy will decrease.

It is becoming obvious that in many people classified as having primary epilepsy, a chemical abnormality exists in the brain, which from time to time allows seizures to occur. It is difficult to study the basic causes of epilepsy because of the inaccessibility of the brain, but it is generally accepted that the chemicals involved in seizure production include the gamma-aminobutyric acid (GABA) system.

Defining the chemicals involved has allowed new drugs to be designed specifically to alter the GABA system. Such drugs include vigabatrin and tiagabine (see Appendix 1).

Secondary Epilepsy

Secondary epilepsy is an easier concept to understand. The seizures are secondary, or subsequent, to some definable abnormality of the brain. Using presently available tests, the abnormality can be detected. The abnormality may have been present at birth, it may be a scar resulting from a subsequent head injury or from meningitis, and so on.

If there is a scar in the brain, the surrounding cells may be distorted and abnormal. Simply look at the tissue around any scar on your body; it appears to be pulled and puckered. If the cells are out of shape, it is possible that they may not function normally. In the case of the brain, such abnormal functions could lead to seizures.

SPECIFIC CAUSES OF EPILEPSY

Inheritance

People with epilepsy often ask if their epilepsy is likely to be handed on to their children, or they are confused as to why epilepsy should suddenly appear in their family, saying, 'No one else in my family has epilepsy.' Not surprisingly, there are many factors involved in assessing the risk of inheritance of epilepsy, making it difficult to predict for specific individuals.

Generally it can be predicted that if one parent has epilepsy, the chances of children developing it are much the same as the population at large, about 1–2 per cent. On the other hand, if both parents have epilepsy, the chances increase to about 10 per cent. It is important to realise that it is not the epilepsy as such that is inherited, but the cause of the epilepsy. In other words, if someone develops epilepsy after a head injury or an operation on the brain, this is not in their genetic make-up and so cannot be handed on.

The past decade has been one of great progress in the study of the genetics of epilepsy, although, while the issues are clearer now than previously, it is still not possible to give genetic advice to most people with epilepsy. The genetics of epilepsy are complex and standard patterns of inheritance are only seen in a small number of cases. The primary generalised epilepsies seem to have a greater tendency to be inherited than do partial seizures. However, one can see very striking family clustering with all of the epilepsies.

Lack of Oxygen to the Brain (Hypoxia)

If for some reason the supply of oxygen to the brain is cut off, damage to the brain cells occurs after a few minutes, which may subsequently lead to the development of seizures. Hypoxia may occur to the foetus during the process of birth. It may occur after a stroke where the blood supply to a particular area of the brain is cut off or in any situation where breathing is interrupted for some time.

Brain Damage and Brain Tumours

Brain damage, which results in scar tissue, predisposes individuals to developing epilepsy. What is often confusing for people is that there may be a long lag period, often years, between the damage occurring and the seizures commencing. The reasons for the delay, and for the seizures eventually commencing, are unknown.

Many people who develop epilepsy fear that it was caused by a brain tumour. Brain tumours are an uncommon cause of epilepsy, especially in children. Nevertheless, it is important to dispel this fear as soon as possible. With the tests available today, reassurance can be given on this matter.

Infections

Epilepsy may arise from damage to the brain resulting from meningitis (bacterial infection), encephalitis (viral infection), infections transmitted from mother to baby during pregnancy (e.g. toxoplasmosis) and parasites such as the sheep tapeworm (*Echinococcus*) or dog tapeworm (*Toxacara*).

SEIZURE-PROVOKING FACTORS

It is important for people with epilepsy and parents of epileptic children to be aware of seizure-provoking factors because, as a general rule, provoked seizures do not respond to an increase in AEDs. It is usually better, if possible, to avoid or modify the trigger factor. Some of these factors include:

Lack of Sleep

It has long been known that sleep deprivation can alter the brain's electrical activity and may provoke fits. These fits are especially common in adolescents and young adults, and lack of sleep is often a major provoking factor in juvenile myoclonic epilepsy (see pp. 53–55). A good night's sleep every night is recommended for all those who have epilepsy. This does not mean that they should never stay up late or become tired, but simply that they need to be sensible.

Menstruation

Some women with epilepsy may have a deterioration in seizure control prior to or during their periods. This is called *catamenial exacerbation of seizures.* (Others may have seizures only in association with their periods. This is called *catamenial epilepsy.*) The cause is unclear, although it seems likely that it relates in some way to hormonal changes. It has been suggested that fluid retention may also be involved, but there is little evidence for this. Also, in some women there may be a fall in the AED blood levels at this time, possibly contributing to an increase in seizure frequency.

Treatment is not entirely satisfactory, with alternatives including the use of clobazam for a few days before and during the period, the use of a diuretic (water tablet) in the same way, increasing the AED dose for a few days during the period or the use of the oral contraceptive pill. None of these approaches is universally helpful, but all are worth considering.

Stress

The relationship between stress and seizure control is difficult to define. What is stressful for one person is not necessarily stressful for the next, and some people are more susceptible to stress than others. Few formal studies have looked at this relationship, but those that have, as well as the reported results of using relaxation therapy, suggest that stress does affect seizure control. This view is strongly supported by hearsay from patients in day-to-day clinical practice.

Once again, this problem does not respond to an increase in medication dosage. In fact, an increase may cause drowsiness, unsteadiness and sometimes confusion, which exacerbates the stress, thereby provoking even more seizures. It is important that epileptics whose seizures are stress-related recognise the relationship, and try to deal with the source of the stress. Often this requires no more than a good chat with an uninvolved person, but may require the help of a counsellor, psychologist or psychiatrist. Relaxation or stress-management courses are very helpful for some individuals.

Alcohol

We all know that alcohol tends to reduce inhibitions and it is also known that it potentially increases the risk of seizures. Binge drinking is especially bad for people with epilepsy and will often lead to seizures during the hangover period. These seizures are more likely to occur if the drinking is coupled with a lack of sleep, as is often the case with adolescents and young adults. Excessive alcohol may not mix well with some of the anticonvulsant medications, making the individual drowsy. People with epilepsy who have current driver's licences should be particularly careful about the combination of alcohol, anticonvulsant medication and driving.

The association between seizures and alcohol does not mean that people with epilepsy should never touch alcohol – they can have the occasional beer, wine or spirits in a modest, sensible social way.

Alcoholics who suddenly stop drinking may have withdrawal seizures. These do not represent epilepsy and should, in the main, not be treated with anti-epileptic medication.

Infections

There is an association between infections and increased frequency of seizures, especially in children and the disabled.

It is common for a child whose seizures have been well controlled to show a sudden deterioration in seizure control when suffering from an infection such as a sore throat or tonsillitis. Fever is usually present, but not invariably. The deterioration in seizure control usually lasts from three days to a week, and does not respond to an increase in AED dosage. It is important for parents and those caring for disabled people to be aware of this association. It is best to concentrate on managing the infection, as there is nothing that can be done about the epilepsy.

Drugs

Some medications can provoke seizures by lowering the seizure threshold. This is not common, and it is not possible to predict in whom this might occur. However, if it has happened to someone on one occasion with the use of a particular medication – for example, pethidine – then it is likely to occur again in the same individual if they receive that drug again. It should thus be avoided. In general, people with epilepsy are told that certain medications or alcohol 'do not mix with their pills'. While this is correct, the concept of certain substances lowering the seizure threshold and increasing the risk of seizures is little discussed. A list of such medications is shown in Table 3.1. If a medication is on this list, it does not mean that someone with epilepsy should never receive it. The implications, however, are that:

- people with epilepsy should be aware that some medicines can lower the seizure threshold; and
- medications that can lower the seizure threshold should only be used if they are really necessary and no suitable alternative exists.

TABLE 3.1 – MEDICATION WHICH MAY LOWER SEIZURE THRESHOLD

MEDICATIONS	RELATIVE FREQUENCY OF SEIZURE PROVOCATION	COMMENTS
Anaesthetic drugs		
enflurane	rare	
isoflurane	rare	
propofol	well described	
Anti-arrhythmics		
lignocaine	uncommon	
mexiletine	rare	• with big intravenous doses
Antibiotics		• probably cannot be avoided
penicillins	} relatively common in high dosage	
cephalosporins		
amphotericin		
imipenem		
Antidepressants		• patients should be informed of risk
tricyclics	uncommon	
selective serotonin re-uptake inhibitors	uncommon	• increased seizures usually occur within 2–6 weeks of starting antidepressant
monoamine oxidase inhibitors	uncommon	
doxepin	rare	
nefazodone	uncommon	
Antihistamines		• widely used and found in many over-the-counter medicines
azatadine		• suggest avoiding unless essential
cyproheptadine	} probably quite rare	• use non-sedating antihistamines in preference
dexchlorpheniramine		
methdilazine		
pheniramine maleate		
promethazine		
Antimigraine		
sumatriptan	rare	

chlorpromazine	uncommon	avoid – if possible
clozapine	common	avoid – if possible
flupenthixol	rare	
fluphenazine	rare	
haloperidol	uncommon	
olanzapine	uncommon	
pimozide	uncommon	
risperidone	uncommon	
thioridazine	uncommon	
thiothixene	uncommon	
trifluoperazine	uncommon	
Bronchodilators		
aminophylline	well described	avoid – if possible
theophylline		
Cough and cold remedies		
triprolidine and pseudoephedrine	probably quite rare	• widely used and found in many over-the-counter medicines
pseudoephedrine		• suggest avoiding unless essential
Hormonal preparations		
oral contraceptives	uncommon	• patients should be warned of risk
hormone replacement therapy	uncommon	• increased seizures occur within 1–4 weeks of starting oral contraceptives or hormone replacement therapy
Immunomodifiers		
cyclosporin	common	
Narcotic analgesics		
pethidine	common	avoid – use morphine
fentanyl	uncommon	avoid – if possible
Stimulant medications		
dexamphetamine	uncommon	• parents/patients should probably be made aware of a quite low risk
methylphenidate	anecdotal reports	

Source: *Australian Prescriber*

Chapter 4

Different Seizure Types

As discussed in Chapter 2, epilepsy consists of, or is made up of, seizures, and can be discussed in terms of:

- *Types of seizures.* A person may have tonic clonic seizures but this does not explain the sort of epilepsy they have, as tonic clonic seizures can occur in several types of epilepsy.
- *Type of epilepsy, or epilepsy syndrome.* A person with a particular syndrome may experience several seizure types as a part of that syndrome. For example, someone with the Lennox-Gastaut Syndrome may have absences, or myoclonic or tonic clonic seizures.

This chapter discusses only the seizure types. The epilepsy syndromes are discussed in the next chapter.

People with epilepsy should be able to define precisely what types of seizures and what type of epilepsy they have. It is not adequate for epileptics to simply say 'I have epilepsy'. They should be able to say, for example, 'I have complex partial seizures', or 'My child has benign partial epilepsy'.

People need to be aware of the nature of their epilepsy for several reasons. Different types of epilepsy have different outlooks and people need to have some idea of what the future holds. Also, if people with epilepsy are adequately informed they can provide correct information to others, including health professionals and the general public. The lay public generally perceives all epilepsy as being represented by tonic clonic convulsions, where the individual falls to the ground in an unconscious state, jerks the limbs and then takes some time to recover. It is vital the message be spread that there are many types of epilepsy and different seizure types, most of which are much less dramatic than tonic clonic seizures. This public education role is being carried out by epilepsy associations but would be greatly strengthened if individuals with epilepsy were more precise in conversation and when filling out various bureaucratic forms about the type of epilepsy they have.

GENERALISED AND PARTIAL SEIZURES

From a practical point of view, seizures can be divided into generalised or partial seizures (see Table 4.1).

A *generalised seizure* implies that abnormal electrical activity involves both halves of the brain (both cerebral hemispheres) from the onset, and is typically associated with loss of consciousness. Myoclonic seizures are the exception to this general rule – they are generalised but consciousness is not always lost.

Partial seizures, on the other hand, start in one cerebral hemisphere, and the abnormal electrical activity remains there rather than spreading to the other side of the brain. While there may be a loss or change of awareness, the individual retains consciousness. Partial seizures may sometimes spread to become generalised. This process is called 'secondary generalisation'. The person commences with a partial seizure, be it complex or simple partial, which progresses to a tonic clonic seizure.

Within these main divisions of generalised and partial seizures there are several different types of seizures, most of which will be discussed in detail in the course of this chapter. Some are mentioned in the table below but not the text, as they are relatively uncommon and do not warrant detailed description.

TABLE 4.1 – THE CURRENT CLASSIFICATION OF SEIZURES

PRESENT CLASSIFICATION	OLD TERMINOLOGY (A)
Generalised seizures **(convulsive or non-convulsive)**	
Tonic clonic seizures	Grand mal
Tonic seizures	Grand mal
Clonic seizures	Grand mal
Atonic (astatic) seizures	Akinetic seizures, or drop attacks
Myoclonic seizures	Minor motor seizures
Absence seizures	Petit mal
– Absences	
– Atypical absences	
Partial seizures	Focal or local seizures

Complex partial seizures
  (consciousness impaired)
  – simple partial onset
  – consciousness impaired
    at onset
	Psychomotor or temporal lobe
	  seizures

Simple partial seizures
  (consciousness not impaired)
  – with motor symptoms
  – with somatosensory or
    special sensory symptoms
  – with autonomic symptoms
  – with psychic symptoms
	
	Jacksonian seizures
	Focal sensory seizures

Partial seizures that secondarily generalise	

(A) While it is hard to break the habit, it is preferable not to use the old terminology.

COMMON GENERALISED SEIZURES

Generalised Tonic Clonic Seizures (GTCS)

Generalised tonic clonic seizures (formerly called grand mal) are a very common type of seizure. Approximately 60 per cent of children with epilepsy will have tonic clonic seizures. These may begin without warning or be preceded by an aura. If the episodes are preceded by an aura, which in itself is a partial seizure, the episodes are then secondarily generalised tonic clonic seizures. These are discussed later in this chapter.

A tonic clonic seizure commences with a sudden loss of consciousness, so if the individual is standing at the time, they will fall to the ground. This is rapidly followed by a general stiffening of the body, which is called the *tonic phase* of the fit. During this time the muscles go quite rigid, and it is for this reason the individual cannot breathe. The face and lips may go blue because of inadequate amounts of oxygen in the blood. (This discolouration is called cyanosis.) Then the *clonic phase*, which consists of jerking of the body, commences. The muscles relax and breathing starts again. As breathing begins, air is pushed through accumulated saliva in the mouth, accounting for the 'frothing at the mouth' of tonic clonic seizures. During the clonic phase the patient may bite their tongue, or pass urine or a motion, although these three events happen less often in children than in adults. The clonic movements gradually settle down and the person becomes relaxed and limp as if exhausted.

The person usually recovers rapidly, but, if the seizure has been prolonged, may go into a deep sleep. While recovering, the individual may feel weak, headachy or fatigued, and sometimes irritable and confused. Depending upon where the seizure has taken place, the person may sustain injuries to the limbs or head.

Most tonic clonic seizures, frightening though they appear, are relatively short-lived, lasting several minutes. Some seizures, however, may be very prolonged, or a number of tonic clonic convulsions may follow each other in rapid succession. The person is then unable to breathe adequately and runs the risk of developing hypoxia (insufficient oxygen to the brain). If a seizure, or a successive run of seizures, has lasted for more than 30 minutes, the situation is called *status epilepticus*. This is a medical emergency and will be discussed later in this chapter.

Do not move the patient, unless the person falls near something dangerous such as a fire.

Do not try to force anything between the teeth.
If you force an object between the teeth, you will break them or get your fingers bitten.
Tongues heal – broken teeth do not!

As soon as the jerking stops and breathing starts, make sure that the patient can breathe freely.
Loosen clothing around the neck and turn the head to the side so that the tongue does not fall back.
(It is impossible to swallow one's tongue as it is firmly fixed to the floor of the mouth.)

Do nothing more! Leave the person to recover.

Do not:

- Slap the face
- Try to 'bring the person round'
- Give anything to drink
- Restrain unless it is absolutely essential

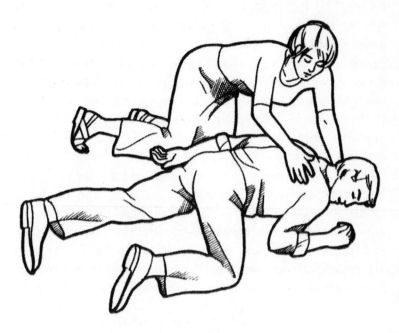

Fig. 4.1 First-aid instructions for tonic clonic seizures

Myoclonic Seizures

Myoclonic seizures are brief, shock-like, involuntary contractions of the muscles that are either rhythmic or sporadic. Often the contractions are symmetrical and involve the muscles of the head and upper limbs. These seizures are sometimes followed by tonic clonic seizures.

We have all experienced myoclonus in the form of the jerking, usually of the legs, that occurs when we are drifting off to sleep. These involuntary movements are called hypnogogic jerks and are quite normal. If, however, this sort of jerking occurs frequently, and is not associated with simply going off to sleep, it is likely that the episodes are myoclonic seizures.

Absence Seizures

Absence seizures (formerly called petit mal) are a form of generalised epilepsy. During such a seizure there is a cessation in mental functioning that begins and ends suddenly. The attacks may last for 1–30 seconds, occasionally longer. They often occur many times a day. The typical features are staring, the eyes drifting upwards and the eyelids flickering. It is quite apparent that the child (as the seizures usually occur in children) is absent ('not with it').

During an absence seizure the individual is unconscious. Recurrent absences will therefore make it difficult for a child to maintain attention and may well have an adverse effect on learning. In fact, it is not uncommon for children with absences to be referred to the doctor with symptoms of inattention and learning difficulties reported from school. The seizures themselves may have gone unnoticed.

Note: The terms 'petit mal' and 'grand mal' are no longer used. *Grand mal*, from the French, implies a 'big sickness', while *petit mal* implies the opposite, namely a 'small sickness'. While absence seizures (petit mal) are certainly much less dramatic than tonic clonic (grand mal) convulsions, and therefore represent 'a smaller sickness', the problem is that 'petit mal' is used to describe anything that is not grand mal in nature. Many adult patients who have complex partial seizures with episodes of staring and being absent will call their seizures 'petit mals'. This confusion accounts for the fact that something like 20–30 per cent of people with epilepsy surveyed state that they have petit mal. This is not the case. The old terminology is imprecise and should not be used.

COMMON PARTIAL SEIZURES

Complex Partial Seizures (CPS)

Complex partial seizures (previously called psychomotor or temporal lobe seizures) are probably the most common type of seizure in all age groups. They arise mainly from the temporal lobes but may also come from the frontal and, less commonly, parietal and occipital lobes.

There are four main groups of causes of complex partial seizures arising from the temporal lobes. First, and most commonly, the cause of the seizures cannot be exactly identified. Secondly, the seizures can arise from a temporal lobe injury, which in turn may have resulted from brain damage from birth, meningitis or a head injury. Thirdly, there may be abnormalities of tissue development in the hippocampal part of the temporal lobe, or small non-malignant tumours. Finally, the seizures can be caused by temporal lobe scarring resulting from *status epilepticus* or prolonged febrile convulsions.

The temporal lobe contains an area called the limbic system in which the heart, blood vessels, respiration and gastro-intestinal systems are represented in terms of function (see Fig. 4.2). This area also deals with smell and memory. Considering the number of functions within the temporal lobe, it is not surprising that the symptoms of complex partial seizures are varied and difficult to diagnose. Quite frequently there are distortions of sensation, which may include strange feelings in the abdomen, odd smells, the hearing of voices or music and sometimes visual hallucinations. A well-known distortion is called the deja vu phenomenon. The person will have a sense that the situation in which they are in is familiar, even though they have never been in that setting before. There may also be disturbances of speech, where the person has difficulty in talking, or says things that are quite inappropriate at the time.

Emotional features including fear or a sense of strangeness, and sometimes physical sensations such as giddiness, may also occur

Complex partial seizures are sometimes preceded by an aura. It is often felt that there is something mystical about an aura, as if it is a warning sent specifically to tell the person that they are going to have a seizure. **In fact, an aura is in itself a simple partial seizure.** In some individuals the aura will proceed no further, while in others it will be followed by a complex partial seizure. This in turn might be followed by secondary generalisation to a tonic clonic seizure.

A person having a complex partial seizure has a fixed stare and shows no awareness of their surroundings. To the outside observer the individual is quite clearly conscious but 'not with it'. The person will often not respond when spoken to, or, if they do, the response may be quite out of context with the question asked. They may also make repetitive movements called automatisms, where they fiddle with their hands or clothes, lick their lips or repeatedly swallow.

Because patients appear not with it or to be 'absent' during these episodes, complex partial seizures are often confused with the absences of absence epilepsy. This in turn leads to the inappropriate use of the term 'petit mal'. Complex partial seizures are more prolonged than true absences and may last for several minutes. As they wear off the individual returns to full consciousness and will almost certainly have no recollection of what occurred during the seizure. The person may, however, be aware that they have had a seizure because they feel light-headed, strange or may have wandered during the episode. In contrast, true absences end very abruptly.

You are invited to read, at the end of this chapter, a description of some of the problems of complex partial seizures as described by a doctor with temporal lobe epilepsy.

Simple Partial Seizures (SPS)

Simple partial seizures (formerly called focal seizures) are quite common in newborn babies, infants and older people. They involve one part or side of the body, the part affected depending upon where the brain abnormality is situated.

The body is represented on the surface of the brain, as shown in Figure 4.2 on the next page. The areas that seem to be most sensitive to stimulation are those representing the index finger, the thumb, the corner of the mouth and the big toe. Thus it is usual for a simple partial seizure to start in one of these areas. It is then likely to spread around that area and involve that side of the body. During the episode consciousness will be retained, unless secondary generalisation occurs and the seizure develops into a tonic clonic episode.

Another type of simple partial seizure is known as an *adversive seizure*. During an episode the head and eyes turn to one side. Sometimes the arm to which they turn is elevated and may twitch.

Status Epilepticus

As already mentioned, *status epilepticus* implies either a prolonged continuous seizure or repeated seizures with incomplete recovery of consciousness. It can be subdivided into two broad categories:

• *Non-convulsive status.* This implies either absence or complex partial *status epilepticus*, during which there are ongoing seizures of either type. Because these are not associated with any form of body movement, the diagnosis may well be delayed. The main presenting features are an alteration of awareness while consciousness is retained, and sometimes behavioural changes. These changes can be subtle and may be missed.

- *Convulsive status.* This implies either simple partial or tonic clonic *status epilepticus.* If it has been going on for more than 30 minutes, it is a medical emergency. An ambulance or medical help should be called at once.

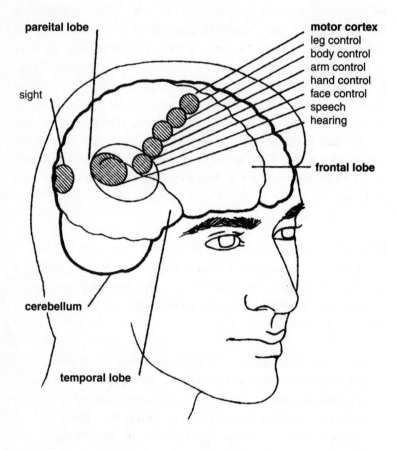

Fig. 4.2 Diagrammatic view of the brain showing some of the areas of body control. Speech is left-sided.

As a general rule, if a seizure lasts as long as 10 minutes, medical or paramedical assistance should be sought. Often by the time the assistance has arrived, the seizure has ceased, but it is better to be overcautious than run the risk of the patient developing hypoxia.

You are now invited to read Dr John Lisyak's description of the problems that he had with the diagnosis of his temporal lobe epilepsy (which commonly involves complex partial seizures), and the impact, both positive and negative, that this had on his life:

My own diagnosis of temporal lobe epilepsy was not made for over a year after the first episode, in spite of quite characteristic complex partial seizures. Several times a day I experienced the sensation of an unusual smell, had feelings of deja vu and later absences when, for a few seconds, I wasn't aware of what I was doing.

Such seizures are fairly common in temporal lobe or complex partial epilepsy. However, what stopped me from even considering such a condition, and what confused the specialists whom I saw, were the feelings that accompanied my turns. It was the feelings that I was most aware of – I didn't even know about the absences. My wife, who had noticed them, thought that they were just an exaggeration of being easily distracted, which I have always been. And the deja vu experiences were not just a simple awareness of something seen before, but a feeling of something strange happening to me, as though for a moment I became part of my surroundings. I would become acutely aware of the shadows and the winter sun and the cold air. They reminded me of something from the past and stood out very vividly; however, I couldn't tell what they meant. Similarly with the 'funny' smell, which was difficult to describe and seemed to be associated with an unusual taste.

But the feeling that accompanied the experience made it worse. Each time I felt restless and fearful, sure that something dreadful was about to happen to me. But then the experience would pass, and I would forget all about it; until next time. This made life confusing, especially just before the diagnosis when such minor seizures were coming several times a day. Eventually I had a major convulsion, which made the diagnosis of epilepsy obvious. Further investigation showed a scar in my right temporal lobe, probably from a difficult birth.

Mixed up with all this was a feeling of helplessness caused by a difficulty with my memory, which seemed to be getting worse and worse. I got to the point of having to work out all my house calls with the help of the street directory, in spite of having worked in the area for some fifteen years and knowing all the patients. Treatment improved things but left me with pockets of lost memory, which interfered with my ability to recall diseases and their treatments. Being in my sixties, I decided to retire.

I had no history of convulsions and there were none in my family. However, like Manning Clark, who also suffered from complex partial seizures, I was searching for answers. Manning called the second volume of his autobiography *The Quest for Grace* – 'A story of my search for wisdom and understanding', or 'How I found my way out of the fog'. I, too, was aware of a kind of fog and searched for answers in religion and other philosophies, in medicine and in writing. As a matter of fact I intended to call the story of my life, if and when I wrote it, *The Quest*, or a name like that. The irony of it is that my search ended with the major convulsion, which forced me to retire but also gave me a new understanding. My further reading about epilepsy taught me that traits such as tenacity, obsessiveness and emotionality, which I have always had, are associated with the epilepsy of the right temporal lobe, where my scar was found.

That was a revelation and produced a kind of elation, which has helped me to face my major crisis and adjust to a completely different way of life. Dostoevsky wrote, 'I want to be there when everyone suddenly understands what it has all been for.' My new insight hasn't made me understand it all, but it has taken away a lot of the stress of constant searching.

It has been said that happiness is a good anticonvulsant. I am convinced that understanding is also, and that the two go together. Prior to my knowing about my epilepsy I can't say that I had led an unhappy life. I had succeeded in a number of fields and I had a happy married life. However, I had always been aware of something missing, something that seemed impossible to define. It wasn't discontentment; it was lack of fulfilment, but why and because of what shortcoming, I could not tell. It was part of the emotional changes that I experienced, which were sometimes extreme, often unpredictable, but usually related to external circumstances – success-producing exhilaration and failure-producing despondency.

All failure was devastating to me. As I was a perfectionist, even the most understandable lack of success produced feelings of hopelessness, and helplessness, which I had to learn to control – through self-suggestion, through positive thinking, and through various methods of deep relaxation and meditation. I know that my interest in psychiatry came from that search.

Understanding does not necessarily change the reactions but it makes a difference to their severity. When it was decided that I go off the tablets because I had had no fits for over three years, I was all right for a few weeks and then suffered another major convulsion. This was followed by the usual depression. However, because of the knowledge I had gained, this depression was not accompanied by feelings of hopelessness. Even the 'funny smell' that returned, together with the emotional dread, wasn't nearly as disturbing because I knew what was happening. Not knowing what is happening to you or how you can be helped is very confusing and demoralising.

Most people who suffer from epilepsy start having convulsions early in life and become aware of being different from an early age. Manning Clark suffered his first convulsion when he was fourteen; however, his mother noticed a difference much earlier in other ways, in him not being able to walk until he was four, for instance. He writes in *The Puzzles of Childhood*:

Each night my mother clings to me: sometimes I think she is crying, and I wonder why. I look up at her from my bed, and see tear-drops on her cheeks, and she says to me, 'I worry sometimes, Mann dear, what's going to happen to you. You're not like the others'.

I have no such memories of my mother, but I do have memories of not being able to do what other children could. The village fair that filled everyone with wonder and excitement made me feel uneasy, and I was never happy to go on a ferris wheel. And in December, on St Nicholas night, I hid under the bed. It wasn't the benign old man with his two or three angels that frightened me, but that other one who came with them. It was Crampus who had horns and a tail that I feared. He carried a basket on his back and I often heard adults say that he'd take children away in that basket if they were naughty.

These early memories help to explain the uncertainty that I felt about myself and how I happened to be searching for answers from such an early age. This search, this quest, became all the more acute after I came to Australia, at the age of twelve, and found my whole life pattern changed. Not only could I not understand or properly relate to other children, but also my family's situation and status changed. In the village everyone knew us and respected us because my grandparents had been mead-makers. In Sydney, in 1936, apart from a few people we had contact with through the Yugoslav Club, no one knew us, or cared to know.

Thus, a combination of external circumstances and those of my internal world brought about some of the loneliest years of my life. My traits of 'tenacity' and 'obsessiveness' enabled me to do well at school, and my conscientious study gave me a way of getting out of the poverty and alienation in which my family found itself. However, 'emotionality', which is also part of right temporal lobe irritation, gave me an intense feeling of isolation. My brother and my friends had left school and were working, while I seemed to be spending most of my life on my own. I didn't find a kindred soul until much later in high school, and searched for outlets in lone bike rides, in reading and listening to music and in religion, all of which meant more hours of loneliness. The effects from these early experiences carried on into my adult life, and never allowed me to be completely free from self-drive or from unexpected feelings of isolation.

Such experiences are not unique to those with epilepsy. Any chronic illness or chronic stress changes our lives and causes unpleasant symptoms. However, it also makes us develop capacities that remain undeveloped in other people. Roslyn Woodward, a psychologist working with people suffering from chronic fatigue syndrome, explains it well in one of her articles. She wrote:

> *Chronic illness ... means you have a chance to reflect, and gain insights and wisdom and knowledge and humour that many people who are fit and healthy don't have a chance to develop.*

Professor Oliver Sacks believes that people suffering from an illness or a handicap can reorganise their lives in order to find undeveloped potential within them – 'liberation through illness'. He refers to a process by which a disaster can be turned into success, 'from disability to new sensibility'. Manning Clark's

45

parents were given such advice in 1929, when he was fourteen years old. Dr Adey told them that his was a:

> ... form of epilepsy which was a common affliction for those with extraordinary imaginations, stormy temperaments, and strange insights into human behaviour. I should think of it not as a badge of infamy, or a handicap, but a gift which I must treasure, and turn to advantage.

Very good advice, and advice that all of us who go through those feelings of worthlessness and hopelessness should be given.

Chapter 5

The Main Types of Epilepsy

The main benefit of classifying epilepsy into syndromes, or grouping individuals with similar types of epilepsy together, is that it allows an assessment of outlook over time (prognosis).

The syndromes discussed in this chapter refer to children rather than adults, because 60–70 per cent of epilepsy commences in childhood and adolescence. Further information on the rarer types of epilepsy should be obtained from a doctor.

The classification of epilepsy is complicated, but it is in part age-related. The four main subgroups are newborn babies, infancy (from one month to one year), childhood, and childhood and adolescence. Table 5.1 shows the syndromes that have been identified in these four subgroups.

It is not possible to discuss all the syndromes in the table in detail, but following are the more common ones.

TABLE 5.1 – EPILEPSY SYNDROMES IN INFANCY, CHILDHOOD AND ADOLESCENCE (A)

In newborn babies
- Benign neonatal convulsions
- Early myoclonic encephalopathy
- Other epileptic syndromes in newborn babies

In infancy and childhood
- Febrile convulsions
- Infantile spasms
- Benign myoclonic epilepsy in infants
- Severe myoclonic epilepsy in infants
- Myoclonic epilepsy in non-progressive encephalopathies
- Epileptic seizures in children with inborn errors of metabolism
- Myoclonic-astatic epilepsy of early childhood
- Lennox-Gastaut Syndrome

In childhood
- Childhood absence epilepsy
- Epilepsy with myoclonic absences
- Epilepsy with generalised convulsive seizures
- Benign partial epilepsy of childhood
- Benign partial epilepsy with centro-temporal spikes
- Benign epilepsy of childhood with occipital spikes
- Benign psychomotor epilepsy
- Landau-Kleffner Syndrome
- Epilepsy with continuous spikes and waves during slow sleep

In childhood and adolescence
- Photosensitive epilepsies
- Juvenile absence epilepsy
- Juvenile myoclonic epilepsy
- Epilepsy with tonic clonic seizures on awakening
- Benign partial seizures of adolescence
- Progressive myoclonic epilepsy in childhood and adolescence
- Reflex epilepsies (especially photosensitive epilepsy)

(A) The classification of syndromes may well change over time, so material presented here may require revision at a later date.

FEBRILE CONVULSIONS

Febrile convulsions occur in about 4 per cent of young children aged six months to five years in association with fever. They may recur in about 30 per cent of children who have had a previous single febrile convulsion. These convulsions are included in the usual list of syndromes, but they do not, in fact, represent epilepsy other than in exceptional circumstances. Seizures that occur in association with fever, but which are due to a brain infection such as meningitis or encephalitis, or that occur in a child with underlying epilepsy, are *not* febrile convulsions.

Febrile convulsions may be very frightening for parents, who quite frequently think their child is dying. This is not the case. Febrile convulsions are essentially harmless. Unless they are recurrent or unusually prolonged, they *never* lead to the subsequent development of epilepsy.

INFANTILE SPASMS

Infantile spasms are a form of myoclonic epilepsy that occur during infancy, usually between three and eight months of age. The spasms consist of sudden symmetrical contractions of muscles and involve both sides of the body. In the most common variety there is a sudden bending of the body, either of the trunk or the neck.

A baby who is lying comfortably will suddenly bring his or her legs up at the hips, throw the arms out and try to lift the head. Often the baby will cry out after a spasm and be rather irritable. This is part and parcel of the seizure and does not indicate any pain. The attacks are repetitive, with each one lasting only a few seconds. Children who can sit at the time of onset of infantile spasms will bend at the waist and put their head between their legs. This movement is called a 'salaam' attack. Attacks (seizures) may be provoked by handling the child and will often occur when the child is drowsy, either just going off to sleep or just having woken. This association with handling, or disturbing, the baby often leads parents to believe that they provoked the seizure. This is not so, but is a source of concern and sometimes guilt for parents.

The diagnosis is made by the combination of the spasms, developmental delay and the findings of hypsarrhythmia (a totally disorganised electroencephalograph, or EEG). This EEG finding is seen in 70–80 per cent of children with infantile spasms.

As a child with this form of epilepsy gets older, the spasms will decrease in frequency. They will, however, be replaced by other seizure types, usually tonic clonic seizures. In addition, there will often be evidence of some degree of mental retardation. The outlook for children with infantile spasms is not good, with only about 30 per cent of affected children ending up physically or mentally normal.

As already suggested, the treatment of this condition is not all that satisfactory, and includes the use of vigabatrin, sodium valproate, steroid medications or nitrazepam. Vigabatrin has the potential problem, when used on a long-term basis, of loss of peripheral vision. However, in view of the serious nature of infantile spasms, it should be tried early on – if it is going to work there should be a response in seven to ten days. If it is not helpful by then, the drug should be withdrawn. The likelihood of any visual damage would be very small. If vigabatrin stops the spasms, which is especially the case with underlying tuberose sclerosis, the benefits may well be seen to outweigh the potential side effect of visual loss, which seems to occur in 10–30 per cent of people exposed to the medication on a long-term basis. There are also surgical possibilities on the horizon.

THE LENNOX-GASTAUT SYNDROME

The Lennox-Gastaut Syndrome usually occurs in preschool-aged children who have previously been quite normal. Some people see it as being similar to infantile spasms, but occurring later in childhood. Indeed, some children with infantile spasms may proceed on to the Lennox-Gastaut Syndrome.

Frequent seizures are the main features of the syndrome. The seizures are mostly tonic and atonic, and atypical absences. The tonic seizures (episodes of going stiff) are usually brief and often occur during sleep. They most commonly involve stiffening of the muscles in the back of the neck, elevation of the shoulders, opening of the eyes and mouth, and temporary cessation of breathing (apnoea). The atonic seizures involve sudden loss of muscle tone and may be preceded by some myoclonic jerks. They often lead to sagging at the knees, head nodding or the individual falling to the ground, usually without loss of consciousness. The absences are like the absences of childhood absence epilepsy, but are called atypical because the EEG findings are not typical of childhood absence epilepsy.

The EEG often shows diffuse, slow spike/waves and runs of rapid spikes during sleep. This is of importance to the neurologist, as it helps with the diagnosis.

Overall, the outlook is poor, with mental retardation developing at, or soon after, the onset of the condition. Some children do not develop retardation, but they are in the minority. The retardation may relate to the underlying cause of the condition, rather than the seizures themselves. Unfortunately, the cause of the Lennox-Gastaut Syndrome is not fully understood. In some children no cause can be found (idiopathic cases), but in the majority there is an underlying brain disorder, often of a quite widespread and diffuse nature. It is hoped that new investigational methods will cast more light on this condition.

The hallmark of the condition is that it is usually quite resistant to regular anti-epileptic medication. Medications of choice include lamotrigine, often combined with sodium valproate, the benzodiazepine group of drugs (nitrazepam, clobazam and clonazepam), steroid medications (ACTH or prednisone), topamax or gabapentin.

PRIMARY GENERALISED EPILEPSY

Primary generalised epilepsy occurs in childhood, and the seizures involve both hemispheres of the brain, as the name implies. The affected child is neurologically and developmentally normal.

Primary generalised epilepsy may be convulsive or non-convulsive and includes the following seizure types:

- Tonic clonic seizures
- Tonic seizures
- Clonic seizures
- Atonic seizures
- Myoclonic seizures
- Absence seizures

Contrary to popular belief, pure absences are quite uncommon, representing about 5 per cent of all childhood epilepsy.

The EEG shows bursts of generalised spike and wave activity in both hemispheres.

BENIGN PARTIAL EPILEPSY WITH CENTRO-TEMPORAL SPIKES

This condition affects 10–20 per cent of children with epilepsy, occurring between two and fourteen years of age, with the peak occurrence at nine years of age.

The main feature is simple partial seizures which mostly occur during sleep, although up to 20 per cent may take place during waking hours. A seizure typically begins in the muscles around the mouth and face, with the child being unable to speak, making a glugging sound, and drooling. The child may experience pins and needles in the area involved and is sometimes able to describe this after the event. Seizure activity may spread to the arm and can involve the whole body in a tonic clonic seizure. Because the seizure onset can pass without notice, onlookers think that the child is having a tonic clonic seizure.

If the episodes are typical, occurring during the night with involvement of the face, as described above, there is no need to do any investigations other than an EEG. The EEG will show epileptic discharges in the centro-temporal area.

The outlook is excellent, with about 98 per cent of patients being seizure-free by twelve years of age and probably all patients by seventeen years of age. The occurrence of seizures in adult life in these children is no more frequent than in the general population.

There is some disagreement as to whether anti-epileptic medication is necessary for these children. However, because some fits occur during the day and some of the night-time fits are prolonged or frightening, most people would suggest treatment. The drug of choice is carbamazepine and it should be continued for two or three years, or until the condition ceases spontaneously, usually at about twelve years of age.

JUVENILE MYOCLONIC EPILEPSY (JME)

Juvenile myoclonic epilepsy has been recognised for some time, but not widely so. It would surprise people to learn that it is almost certainly more common than childhood absence epilepsy, for example, which is regarded by many doctors and people with epilepsy as occurring frequently. This condition starts in adolescence, usually between twelve and eighteen years of age. It may, however, start in late childhood or in adult life.

The main features are myoclonus (muscular jerking), particularly in the mornings during the first hour or two after waking. At this time the person is shaky and clumsy, and may drop things. Early morning shakiness may be present for a long time before the first major seizure, which brings the condition to light. When asked about any past medical history, the person often doesn't mention the early morning shakiness or jumpiness, as they have come to regard this as part and parcel of themselves, saying, 'I am not a morning person' or, 'I am no good before 10 am'.

Most people with this condition present with tonic clonic seizures, which tend to occur after waking in the mornings and are often preceded by a flurry of myoclonic jerks. The myoclonus and tonic clonic seizures may be precipitated by photic (light) stimulation, a lack of sleep, and alcohol. Absences may also occur in juvenile myoclonic epilepsy.

As far as tests are concerned, the EEG shows a pattern of fast spike and wave and/or polyspike and wave discharge, which may help the neurologist in making the diagnosis.

Juvenile myoclonic epilepsy is not associated with any abnormality of intellect, but there appears to be a quite strong genetic component. This means that the condition may be handed to future generations, although the exact mode of inheritance is not clear. It appears to be a lifelong condition.

Sodium valproate is the drug of choice, as it controls both the myoclonus and the tonic clonic seizures in the majority of cases. The withdrawal of medication is usually associated with a recurrence of seizures, as the condition is permanent. This implies the need to take medication for life. For those individuals who might develop side effects from sodium valproate and thus find its use unacceptable, lamotrigine is often a very suitable alternative, with other possibilities being sulthiame or clobazam. It is important for individuals with juvenile myoclonic epilepsy to avoid sleep deprivation, especially in association with alcohol ingestion, as these are powerful seizure-provoking factors in this condition.

REFLEX EPILEPSY

Reflex epilepsy is triggered by some form of sensory stimulus. There are many types of reflex epilepsy, but the most common is *photosensitive* epilepsy.

There are two forms of photosensitivity: a photosensitive trait (tendency), and photosensitive epilepsy. The first can be identified in some individuals during an EEG. When lights are flashed at them, they show epileptic activity, but do not necessarily have a seizure. Other individuals, however, not only show the EEG abnormality, but also have seizures provoked by light. Such people have photosensitive epilepsy.

Photosensitive epilepsy is usually manifested by tonic clonic seizures, which may sometimes be preceded by myoclonus. Absences may also occur but are uncommon.

Flickering light such as strobe lights, car headlights, alternating dark and shade created, for example, by an avenue of trees, or the reflection from sunlight on water can provoke a seizure. Although watching television itself is not a problem, if the child sits too close to the set or approaches it to change channels, the background flickering of the screen may be a stimulus to a seizure. This also applies to computer video games, but not to standard office video display units.

Photosensitivity can be well managed by avoiding the provoking factor as much as possible, wearing sunglasses and, if necessary, the use of sodium valproate or lamotrigine.

Chapter 6

How is Epilepsy Diagnosed?

There are a number of tests used to assist in making a diagnosis of epilepsy, but these are often not absolutely diagnostic by themselves. This chapter will discuss some of the investigations that a doctor may suggest.

CLINICAL HISTORY

Despite all the advances in technology, the most vital aid to making a diagnosis of epilepsy remains the story given by the patient, the patient's relatives or other observers. While it is recognised that descriptions of the seizures are not always accurate, as in the heat of the moment things can be forgotten or misinterpreted, an eyewitness account is of great value. In taking the patient's history, it is important for the doctor to obtain information about the patient's birth, subsequent illnesses and whether anyone else in the family has epilepsy. It is also often of value to the doctor to obtain information about any events that may have preceded the seizure, such as a series of late nights, excessive alcohol intake, abnormally severe stress, and so on.

PHYSICAL EXAMINATION

All patients with epilepsy should have a full physical examination the first time they present to their doctor. In primary epilepsy – that is, where no cause can be found – the physical examination will usually be normal. On the other hand, if the epilepsy is caused by an established brain problem such as a head injury or cerebral palsy, abnormalities of the nervous system may well be found on physical examination.

LABORATORY TESTS

It may be appropriate to measure, at least in association with an initial seizure, the blood concentrations of sugar, calcium, magnesium and, very occasionally, amino acids. It may also be desirable to look at the chromosome pattern, as some genetic conditions, especially those associated with mental retardation such as the Fragile X Syndrome, may be associated with seizures. In some circumstances, a lumbar puncture, which means obtaining a sample of spinal fluid, may be required. This is not, however, a routine investigation in epilepsy.

ELECTROENCEPHALOGRAPHY (EEG)

The EEG measures differences in electrical activity between different parts of the brain arising from the spontaneous activity of the brain cells. There are a number of different forms of EEG. As this is a very common test used in epilepsy, both for diagnosis and, to a lesser extent, to assess progress once treatment has been commenced, it will be discussed in some detail.

The Routine EEG

A routine EEG involves the patient going to an EEG laboratory where electrodes are placed on the scalp and connected to an electrical recorder. Routine recordings are made with the patient either sitting or lying down. While the recording takes place it is important that the individual remains still. Any muscular movement may be recorded on the EEG tracing and will make it harder to interpret. Keeping still can be difficult for children, and it may take an hour or more to get a satisfactory recording from a child.

The EEG is generally regarded as the mainstay in the diagnosis of epilepsy. While this may be true, the EEG does have some very real limitations. These include the fact that it may be technically difficult to obtain an adequate recording in a young child. More important is the fact that the patterns appearing on an EEG are often non-specific. The tracing might imply that all is not quite right, but it does not provide precise information as to the nature of the problem. An EEG is generally recorded over a short period of time, perhaps 20–30 minutes, so it may be quite normal at the time it is done for a person who has only occasional seizures. About 35 per cent of patients with epilepsy have a normal EEG during a single recording, and about 20 per cent of non-epileptic people show some abnormality on an EEG when it is done randomly. This does not mean the EEG is not a test worth doing, but simply that it rarely 'makes the diagnosis' except in a few specific types of epilepsy. The results of the EEG need to be interpreted in conjunction with the clinical history of the patient and his or her description of the seizures.

The advantages of the EEG are that it is painless, a relatively short test, and inexpensive. In some forms of epilepsy, such as infantile spasms, the Lennox-Gastaut Syndrome, childhood absence epilepsy and benign partial epilepsy of childhood, it is often very helpful in actually making the diagnosis. The EEG also provides a permanent record that can sometimes be used at a later date to evaluate progress.

A variation on the routine EEG is a sleep-deprived EEG. This is carried out by either keeping the individual awake very late at night or getting them up early in the morning so that when they have their EEG they will be tired and fall asleep. Sleep accentuates EEG abnormalities and can make the test more worthwhile.

Special EEG Studies

It is sometimes necessary to do more sophisticated EEG studies involving a process called telemetry, which is usually carried out under video observation. Occasionally the seizures are simply recorded electrically in the equivalent of a little tape recorder attached to the person's belt. Usually, however, seizures are recorded by video-EEG telemetry, where electrodes are kept on the scalp for days, sometimes weeks, while the person is observed with a video camera. This allows both visual and electrical observation of the seizures.

Such a test would not be done on a routine basis, but certainly has a role to play in the management of difficult epilepsies (where seizure control is poor), where surgery is being contemplated or where pseudo-epileptic seizures might be suspected.

Computerised Tomography (CT Scanning)

During this procedure the person lies with their head in an X-ray machine. A rapid sequence of X-rays of the skull and brain is taken and then repeated after the injection of some dye. This is a painless procedure, other than the injection, but some young children might be a little scared by all the machinery. As there is a need to lie quite still during the procedure to get adequate pictures, a very young child may need to be sedated or given a light general anaesthetic.

CT scanning is useful for excluding the presence of large brain lesions, but in the investigation of epilepsy it has been largely replaced by magnetic resonance imaging (MRI).

MAGNETIC RESONANCE IMAGING (MRI)

As far as the patient is concerned, an MRI scan is similar to a CT scan, except that the whole body goes into the machine, as opposed to just the head, and the MRI is quite noisy. As a general rule, people with primary generalised epilepsy do not require a scan, as there is very rarely any structural brain abnormality. However, those with partial seizures or symptomatic generalised epilepsies should undergo an MRI scan at some stage.

SINGLE PHOTON EMISSION COMPUTERISED TOMOGRAPHY (SPECT)

This is a nuclear medicine test where a radioactive isotope is injected during a seizure. Because of the increased blood flow in the area of brain involved in the seizure, the isotope will be deposited in that area. Subsequent scanning may determine the origin of the seizure. This is a test that is used particularly in the investigation of complex partial seizures with a view to epilepsy surgery.

POSITRON EMISSION TOMOGRAPHY (PET SCANNING)

An injection of a radioactive tracer allows an assessment of brain metabolism. Between seizures, focal areas from which seizures arise have diminished blood flow (a cold spot on the scan), and during seizures they have increased blood flow (a hot spot on the scan). PET scans are mainly used to look for localising evidence in the investigation of people who may be suitable for epilepsy surgery. There is also a significant research role for PET scanning which, over time, should allow a better understanding of brain metabolism and function.

HOW MANY TESTS ARE NECESSARY?

As you can see, there are a large number of tests available in the investigation of epilepsy. The question arises as to how many investigations any one individual might need. The answer will depend on the type of epilepsy and its severity. It is worth mentioning the comments made by Nial O'Donahue, a noted paediatric neurologist, in *Epilepsies of Childhood*:

> At all times the physician should resist the mania for modern investigation. This is always expensive and time consuming and frequently in the worst interests of the patient. There are no 'routine' investigations; there are only those that are indicated by the specific diagnosis presented by the patient.

This comment is as valid today as it was in 1979, perhaps even more so, as there are more tests available now than there were then. From a patient's point of view, it is important to ask why the test is being done and how the result will affect either the diagnosis of epilepsy or management of the condition.

Chapter 7

The Management
of Epilepsy

The term 'management' is used expressly rather than 'treatment', implying that while the use of medication as treatment for epilepsy is essential, the overall management of the condition involves more than taking tablets. There are a number of psychosocial factors that need to be taken into account, such as ensuring that the patient gets sufficient sleep, avoids excessive alcohol, takes their medication regularly and reports any drug side effects to their doctor. Stress is a common seizure-provoking factor and there is a need for this to be discussed openly between patient and doctor.

The accepted forms of management for epilepsy include medical treatment using anti-epileptic medications, surgery, and behavioural (stress) management. More controversial options included hypnosis, naturopathy, acupuncture and dietary management.

MEDICAL TREATMENT

About 70–75 per cent of people with epilepsy will achieve good seizure control with the use of anti-epileptic medications, while about 25 per cent will not respond well to AEDs. These figures probably remain much the same despite the advent of quite a few new medications over the past decade. New medications have provided a greater choice of treatment, some with fewer side effects than the older drugs, but they are probably all much the same in terms of achieving seizure control.

Achieving a Balance

From a practical point of view, *the treatment of epilepsy with medication consists of a balance between seizure control on the one hand and medication side effects on the other.* Most people with epilepsy are aware of how many seizures they have and can report that information to their doctor. At the same time, they are likely to be aware of any side effects from their medication, and once more should discuss these with their doctor. It is this information that is required to find an appropriate balance in the management of epilepsy.

How Much Medication is Necessary?

Some 60–75 per cent of people with epilepsy who achieve control with AEDs require only one medication. This is called *monotherapy*. Others will need more than one AED, but rarely more than two. When a person first starts on anticonvulsant medication, the dose should be increased relative to seizure frequency. There should be no need to add another medication unless the fits are not controlled (assuming that the patient is really taking the medication), or side effects from the drug arise.

Most AEDs need to be taken only twice a day. Some drugs, such as phenytoin, can be taken once a day. There may be times when it is necessary to administer AEDs three times a day, but these are rare. It is often the midday dose that is forgotten or not taken to avoid embarrassment either at school or at work.

Should All Seizures be Treated or Eradicated?

Epilepsy, probably more than most other conditions, requires individualised management. As we have seen, it comes in a variety of forms and different degrees of severity. While it is very tempting to try to control all seizures in every patient, this may be difficult to do, and some individuals may pay a high price in terms of drug side effects. Once again, it comes back to the balance between seizure control and suffering from drug side effects.

It is essential that agreement is achieved between doctor and patient (or parents/carers) about the degree of seizure control. The emphasis should be on what is desired by the patient, not necessarily on what is seen as desirable by the doctor. It is, after all, the patient's right to decide upon the degree of seizure control they want, provided the person accepts the responsibilities imposed on them by having seizures. It is not the prerogative of the doctor to insist on complete eradication of seizures, particularly if this would be associated with significant drug side effects that may affect quality of life.

Compliance with Medication

The term 'compliance' means adherence to the doctor's instructions, in this instance with regard to medication. People who do not take their medication regularly are called 'noncompliant'. Noncompliance is quite common, and various studies suggest that it occurs in 30–50 per cent of people with epilepsy on an occasional basis.

The traditional medical interpretation on noncompliance is that these patients are 'naughty', irresponsibly ignoring medical advice. An alternative viewpoint is that in some regards noncompliance is normal behaviour in as much as taking medication on a regular basis can be deemed to be abnormal, unless there is very good reason for doing so. The taking of medication is also tedious, and normal forgetfulness means that people will be noncompliant from time to time. Some patients state that they have been noncompliant because of drug side effects, while others may have quite infrequent seizures and have consequently decided it was not worth taking medication regularly to prevent such occasional episodes.

In general terms, though, patients should be encouraged to be compliant. If they are not, the reasons should be sought and discussed fully.

There is, of course, a social responsibility for people with epilepsy to take their medication regularly, particularly if they are in a place of employment where having a seizure could be hazardous to themselves or to others, and if they drive a motor vehicle.

The Management of a Single Seizure

By definition, a single seizure does not constitute a diagnosis of epilepsy, which implies having recurrent unprovoked seizures. As a result, only certain individuals would be required to take anti-epileptic medication after a single seizure.

For example, for individuals with underlying brain damage, or for older people, it is known that the recurrence rate after a single seizure might be in the region of 80–90 per cent. It could be argued that, as the chances of a recurrence are so high, rather than wait for another seizure to occur it might be better to commence treatment after the first episode. It is yet to be proven, however, that such an approach is effective. Individuals whose initial seizure is either very severe or occurs in a situation where there is an associated injury may also be required to commence treatment immediately with an anti-epileptic medication.

Choice of Medication

Medications used in the treatment of the various types of epilepsy that have been discussed will vary according to seizure type and the nature of the epilepsy itself. Some drugs are better for certain seizure types than others, but few of the AEDs are specific for any one seizure type. There is therefore often a choice of AEDs for use in any one person. Again, the choice needs to take into account a balance between likely efficacy on the one hand and side effects on the other.

Tonic Clonic Seizures

AEDs of choice would include carbamazepine, sodium valproate and lamotrigine. Less favoured drugs might include phenytoin, the barbiturates and clonazepam because of their side effects. Others worthy of consideration include clobazam, topiramate and sulthiame.

Tonic Seizures

Tonic seizures, which frequently arise while the person is asleep, are often very resistant to medication. Medications of choice are sodium valproate, lamotrigine, nitrazepam, clonazepam, sulthiame and topiramate.

Myoclonic Seizures

These may occur in individuals who are neurologically and developmentally normal, as well as in people who have neuro-developmental problems. In the latter group, myoclonic seizures are usually more difficult to control. The drugs of choice are sodium valproate, lamotrigine, clobazam, nitrazepam, clonazepam, sulthiame and topiramate. It should be noted that some of the medications used mainly for the treatment of partial seizures can occasionally make myoclonic and absence seizures worse; these include carbamazepine, gabapentin, tiagabine, vigabatrin and possibly levetiracetam.

Absence Seizures

The drug of choice for absence seizures is sodium valproate, with lamotrigine and ethosuximide being alternatives. In patients with atypical absences, where treatment is more difficult, there may be a need to look at other medications, such as clobazam, clonazepam or topiramate. As mentioned under 'Myoclonic Seizures' on the previous page, some medications can occasionally make absence seizures worse.

Complex Partial Seizures

The medications of choice are carbamazepine, lamotrigine, sodium valproate, clobazam and topamax. Other drugs that should also be considered include sulthiame, levetiracetam gabapentin, phenytoin, the barbiturates and tiagabine.

Simple Partial Seizures

Carbamazepine is the drug of choice. Other suitable medications include lamotrigine, sodium valproate, clobazam, levetiracetam, gabapentin, topamax and sulthiame.

Status Epilepticus

As has already been mentioned (see pages 39–41), *status epilepticus* is a medical emergency. Professional help should be sought, and usually the individual will be taken to hospital where anti-convulsant medication will be administered intravenously (into a vein). The possibilities for management of this situation at home are limited. However, in children who recurrently have severe or prolonged seizures, it may well be appropriate for a parent/carer to administer rectal diazepam (Valium) to the individual. This can be done by drawing up some diazepam into a narrow syringe, inserting it into the child's rectum (back passage) and injecting the solution. Not all parents/carers wish to do this, but it will often help to avoid a number of trips to hospital. Midazolam may be a suitable alternative and can be administered into the nose, under the tongue or intramuscularly.

Infantile Spasms

Probably the drug of first choice is vigabatrin, as it either works very well, or not at all, in a few days. It is particularly useful if there is underlying tuberose sclerosis. If it has not worked in seven to ten days, the drug should be abandoned. Alternatives include nitrazepam, steroids such as prednisone or ACTH, lamotrigine or sodium valproate. When the spasms come under control, other seizure types are likely to occur, which require treatment in their own right.

Lennox-Gastaut Syndrome

As for infantile spasms, this form of epilepsy is difficult to manage. The options are similar to those for infantile spasms. Vigabatrin has little role to play in this condition, but topiramate should be considered.

Reflex Epilepsy

It is not always necessary to use drug therapy in reflex epilepsy as it may be possible to prevent the seizures by avoiding the triggering factor. As mentioned (see page 55), the most common form of reflex epilepsy is photosensitive epilepsy, and episodes can be avoided by wearing polarised sunglasses, if the photosensitivity is induced by sunlight, or by sitting some 3 metres away from the television in a well-lit room, if it is related to television watching. If medication is required, sodium valproate or lamotrigine are the drugs of choice. Occasionally, clobazam or clonazepam need to be considered.

Practical Advice about Anti-epileptic Medications

1. If you are taking anti-epileptic drugs (AEDs), do not take any other medications without asking your doctor or chemist. It is safe to take paracetamol for fever or headache, and antibiotics (except erythromycin, if you are on regular carbamazepine) for infections. If you are taking the contraceptive pill, let your doctor know which one – some AEDs make the pill less effective and it may be necessary to try a different pill or a different form of contraception.
2. Avoid alcohol in anything more than social amounts. It does not mix well with AEDs and may trigger fits.
3. Never stop taking AEDs suddenly. This could produce a marked increase in the number of your fits.
4. Do not allow yourself to run out of medication. Always keep a spare prescription at home or with your chemist.
5. If you miss one dose, do not take a double dose of medication to catch up; just get back into your regular dosage routine.
6. For convenience, take your medication with meals. If you are taking several different AEDs, take them all at the same time – once, twice or three times a day as directed.
7. Always keep medications in a locked cupboard away from children.

Drug Monitoring

Doctors will often take blood samples from patients who have epilepsy to measure the concentration of the AED in their blood. Therapeutic drug monitoring determines whether the patient's blood level is within what is called 'the therapeutic range'. This is the range of blood concentrations of AEDs within which most people with epilepsy will have good seizure control with minimum drug side effects. Not all patients have to be within the therapeutic range. Some people may have mild epilepsy and will be well controlled below the therapeutic range, while others who might have more severe seizures will need to have higher blood levels to achieve control.

Measuring AED levels in the blood can be useful, particularly with a drug such as phenytoin, which is handled in a somewhat unusual way in the body. It may occasionally be useful to measure the blood levels of carbamazepine and the barbiturates. There is, however, not much if any value in measuring the blood levels of any of the other AEDs, as there is little relationship between the concentration of AEDs and seizure control.

For some time, the measurement of AED levels in blood was regarded as routine. This attitude persists up to a point, but measurement seems to be practised somewhat less than it was a few years ago. Again, the issue is achieving a balance between seizure control and drug side effects. There are no indications for routine blood-level monitoring in day-to-day clinical practice. The indications for blood-level monitoring include:

- *Poor seizure control.* This may occur because the individual is not taking their medication (noncompliance), is not receiving a sufficient dose or is taking an inappropriate medication. It could also be that the fits are, in fact, uncontrollable, or that the diagnosis of epilepsy is incorrect.
- *Polytherapy (taking more than one medication).* Where seizures have been difficult to control with one drug only and a further medication has been added, there may be interactions between the drugs, and sometimes measurement of blood levels is helpful.
- *Side effects.* If a patient is on one drug only (monotherapy) and suffers from side effects, there

would be little need to measure the blood levels. The side effects could only be caused by the one drug and are likely to be dose-related. If, on the other hand, the patient is on polytherapy, it may not be possible to know which drug is causing the problem. Measuring the blood levels may be helpful in this situation.

- *Epilepsy in very young children, older people or disabled people.* In the first two groups, anticonvulsant medications may be handled differently in the body from the way they are handled in other age groups. For this reason, there may be a role for blood-level monitoring. Also, it may not be possible for the disabled individual to describe their side effects, and it may therefore be helpful to measure blood levels if side effects are suspected.

SURGERY

A small number of people may be helped by surgery, particularly those with complex partial seizures of temporal lobe origin who have not responded to AEDs. There are a number of forms of surgery, including:

- *Temporal lobe surgery.* This is the most commonly performed and successful surgical operation for epilepsy. It will not be discussed in detail here except to say that in appropriately selected individuals with complex partial seizures the results are frequently very good, with 60–70 per cent of people becoming seizure-free post-operatively while still taking an anticonvulsant medication. This form of surgery is only useful if the fits cannot be controlled by medication and if the fits are localised to one side of the brain in the front part of the temporal lobe.

- *Corpus callosotomy.* This operation is sometimes done in individuals with tonic or atonic seizures, particularly those who injure themselves when falling during these seizures. It consists of separating one brain hemisphere from the other. This changes generalised seizures into less severe partial seizures. While this operation sounds drastic, it results in remarkably few side effects and is helpful in some well-chosen individuals.
- *Hemispherectomy.* This is a major surgical procedure used in only the most exceptional circumstances – in infants and very young children with totally uncontrollable seizures. It necessitates removing most of one half of the brain. It will often stop the seizures, but may leave the child with residual weakness of one side of the body. Often the part of the brain removed is found to be abnormal anyway.
- *The removal of a tumour (benign or malignant).* This is not truly epilepsy surgery, as the tumour would require removal in its own right irrespective of the seizures.

BEHAVIOURAL MANAGEMENT

Many individuals with epilepsy have seizures that are related to stress and lifestyle. Generally, these seizures will not respond to the addition of more anti-epileptic medication. Indeed, increasing the dosage will frequently make the individual drowsy and more stressed, which in turn will provoke further seizures, leading to a vicious circle.

Stress-related seizures need to be treated by looking at the causes of the stress and trying to deal with those factors. Relaxation therapy, group therapy and stress management are all overlapping approaches that may be useful and should be considered.

MORE CONTROVERSIAL OPTIONS

With the growing concern about chemicals in the environment, and thus the taking of medications, it is quite common for people with epilepsy to enquire about non-drug treatment options. These include:

Hypnosis

The majority of people would find little place for hypnosis in the management of epilepsy. An exception might be the patient who has a very long aura prior to a seizure. During the aura the patient might be able to use self-hypnosis to prevent the seizure. Unfortunately, auras rarely last long enough for this to be an option.

Naturopathy

Naturopaths have suggested that epilepsy is due to a deficiency of the B group of vitamins. Administering supplements has met with some success in cases of absence epilepsy, but not in other forms of epilepsy.

Acupuncture

The role of acupuncture in the management of epilepsy remains controversial. Acupuncturists see epilepsy as a liver problem, as they believe the liver controls muscular rigidity. There is no conclusive evidence that acupuncture helps people with epilepsy

Dietary Management

Parents frequently ask if epilepsy is related to diet and whether supplementation with vitamins would be helpful. The answer to this is almost certainly 'no'. There have been reports of low blood levels of zinc in association with some of the anti-epileptic medications such as phenytoin and sodium valproate, but zinc supplementation does not improve seizure control. Some patients who have taken phenytoin or the barbiturates on a long-term basis may be folate deficient. With some people, supplementation with folic acid can increase seizure control, but with others it may produce a deterioration in seizure control, so there is no conclusive evidence of its effectiveness.

For patients with severe myoclonic epilepsy or infantile spasms who have failed to respond to medication, the use of a ketogenic (high fat) diet is sometimes recommended. This diet acts by increasing the blood concentration of a variety of acids in the body to produce chemical changes in the brain. This supposedly reduces the tendency for brain cells to discharge, and prevents the spread of discharges within the brain. There is some reported success with the ketogenic diet, but overall the results are disappointing.

Chapter 8

Women and Epilepsy

There are a number of issues that pertain specifically to women who have epilepsy, the most obvious, of course, being pregnancy.

CATAMENIAL EPILEPSY

It has long been recognised that there may be a relationship between the menstrual cycle and seizures. This takes two forms: seizures that occur solely in association with menstruation (catamenial epilepsy), and those that occur more frequently in association with menstruation (catamenial exacerbation of seizures). The latter is much more common than the former. There may also be an exacerbation of seizures at the time of ovulation. It is difficult to ascertain how commonly these associations occur. While they are frequently reported, when patients are asked to keep a record of their seizures relative to their menses, the association is often not as regular as they thought it to be.

It is not clear why menstruation exacerbates seizures (although there is clearly a hormonal relationship), so the management of catamenial epilepsy can be difficult. The approaches include the use of an AED such as clobazam for several days prior to and during the period. This means that the drug is taken for about seven to ten days of the month in addition to the existing anticonvulsant medication. If this is not helpful, it might be worth looking at the use of a water tablet (diuretic), taken on the same days. The third alternative is the use of an oral contraceptive agent.

INTERACTION OF AEDs AND ORAL CONTRACEPTIVES

Many of the anti-epileptic medications will cause the liver to break down the oral contraceptive pill in the body more rapidly than usual, a process called induction. AEDs that do this include carbamazepine, phenytoin, the barbiturates and probably topiramate. This does not mean that women taking the oral contraceptive pill should not take inducing drugs; rather, they would need to be on a high-dose pill instead of a low-dose pill, or use some other form of contraception.

PREGNANCY

There are five issues that are of concern to women with epilepsy with regard to getting pregnant:

- What is the possibility of handing epilepsy on to their children?
- Will the frequency of their seizures increase during pregnancy?
- Will it be safe for the baby if they take anti-epileptic medication during pregnancy?
- What problems will these drugs cause for the newborn baby after birth?
- Will it be possible to breastfeed the infant?

Inheritance of Epilepsy

If one or both parents have epilepsy, the risk of handing it on to their children is up to five times greater than that in the general population. If the parents have epilepsy of an acquired nature, such as after a head injury or following an operation, there is no risk of handing it on to their children.

Seizure Control During Pregnancy

Approximately one-third of women with epilepsy will show no change in seizure control during pregnancy, a further one-third will show an improvement and may well become seizure-free, and the remaining one-third will show a deterioration in seizure control. The deterioration usually occurs in the first three months of pregnancy, with only 1–2 per cent of women with epilepsy having seizures during labour. While this information is generally accepted, the difficulty is in predicting in whom there is likely to be a deterioration in seizure control. As a general rule, women who have more than one tonic clonic seizure a month are those most likely to have a deterioration in seizure control during pregnancy.

Why this deterioration occurs is not certain, although in some individuals there is a fall in blood levels of AEDs as they put on weight during pregnancy. This, however, cannot be the entire explanation, as most individuals will show a deterioration of seizure control in the first three months of pregnancy before there is any significant weight gain. In addition, those individuals whose seizure control improves often have lower blood levels of AEDs as well.

There are two approaches to the measurement of AED blood levels during pregnancy. As AED blood levels almost always fall during pregnancy, one view is that they should be measured in each pregnancy, and drug doses increased irrespective of seizure control. The alternative view is that while AED blood levels may fall, this may not always be associated with a deterioration in seizure control. This view implies that AED blood levels should be measured only if seizures occur, and the drug dose adjusted accordingly. It is not suggested that either view is right or wrong – the patient should discuss her situation with her doctor.

Effect of AEDs on Foetus

The main concern for parents is whether the AEDs can cause harm to the unborn baby. It is known to most women with epilepsy that this is a potential hazard. The process by which AEDs produce abnormalities in the baby is known as teratogenesis. Many of the abnormalities, such as a rather broad bridge of nose and tapered fingers, are relatively minor. There may, however, be heart defects, a cleft palate, mild mental retardation and, of more concern, abnormalities of the nervous system, including spina bifida and anencephaly.

Physical and mental abnormalities have been reported in the offspring of mothers on all the commonly used anti-convulsant medications. The frequency of malformations is two to three times greater in the offspring of women taking AEDs than in the offspring of epileptic women not taking such medications. Poor seizure control and multiple medications are associated with a risk of foetal abnormalities for about 11 per cent. Spina bifida has been reported with all the anticonvulsant medications to date, but particularly with sodium valproate. The risk of spina bifida with sodium valproate is somewhere in the region of 1–2 per cent. Spina bifida and anencephaly can usually be detected by ultrasound at twelve to fourteen weeks of pregnancy. At this stage not a great deal is known about the effects of the new anti-epileptic medications during pregnancy, although when they were studied in animals no abnormalities were noted.

It has been recommended that women with epilepsy take folic acid for one month before conception and three months thereafter, to try to reduce the rate of central nervous system abnormalities. This is good advice but may not always be practical, as more than one-half of women with epilepsy first present to a doctor when they are already about six weeks pregnant.

In summary, although the teratogenetic effect of anti-convulsants needs to be taken into consideration, the risks of stopping treatment – especially the possibility of *status epilepticus* – are probably greater than the risk of having an abnormal infant. Therefore it is appropriate to continue anticonvulsant treatment throughout pregnancy with the assistance of occasional blood level measurements where this is necessary.

Effects of AEDs on Newborn Baby

Anticonvulsants taken by the mother during pregnancy may have some impact on the baby immediately after birth, as they are transmitted across the placenta. Possible effects include drowsiness and a mild bleeding tendency, which responds to vitamin K. Drowsiness is seen particularly in the offspring of women who are taking barbiturates or the benzodiazepine drugs, notably clonazepam. The infants may also show features of a withdrawal reaction with irritability, jitteriness and poor sucking. None of these features is common or serious.

Breastfeeding

All the anti-epileptic medications appear in breast milk to some extent. At worst, they may produce mild drowsiness in the infant. There is no reason for mothers with epilepsy not to breastfeed if they wish to do so. If the mother is concerned that she might have a seizure and drop the baby while breastfeeding, it would seem practical for her to sit on the floor at these times.

Chapter 9

Epilepsy in Children, Older People and Disabled People

This chapter looks at some aspects of epilepsy that pertain more to children, older people and disabled people, especially from a social point of view.

CHILDREN WITH EPILEPSY

Epilepsy has an impact on families because most epilepsy, probably 60–70 per cent, commences in childhood or adolescence.

For parents, the news that their child has epilepsy often provokes a protective response towards their 'wounded' offspring. They may also experience considerable anger and guilt associated with some degree of denial of the epilepsy. Some parents, especially fathers, see their child as having become 'imperfect', leading to a sense of shame and some degree of rejection of the child. All these reactions are normal, representing grief over the apparent loss of the child's health.

From a medical point of view, it is important that these reactions be recognised and discussed as openly as possible.

Following the diagnosis of epilepsy, the child will often react with anger, which is manifested by behavioural change. This is exemplified by a nine-year-old girl whose mother has epilepsy. When the girl was diagnosed with complex partial seizures, and before medication was commenced, her behaviour underwent a profound change. The girl became aggressive and began using abusive language, largely directed at her mother who 'gave her epilepsy'. Even without a parent with epilepsy, this sort of reaction may occur and needs to be dealt with as a matter of urgency. Most children, and adults, who react this way need the opportunity to discuss their feelings (usually fears) openly and regularly. With time the reaction will settle down.

Parents are often anxious about what will happen when their child goes to school. It is easy to say to parents, 'Let him or her lead a normal life', but for parents to be able to stand back and do this is often very difficult. They wonder whether it is true that children with chronic diseases are teased at school, and whom they should tell about their child's epilepsy and medication. The means of coping with epilepsy in a school-aged child varies from family to family, depending on the nature of the school the child is attending, the teachers who are there, and parental expectations. Most teachers are appreciative of information on epilepsy, and such information is available from epilepsy associations.

If a child has a seizure in the classroom, it may be of value for the teacher to do two things. First, note what is happening and report that to the parents or doctor. Secondly, use the episode as a chance to explain to other children in the class what seizures are, as well as showing how the child recovers fully from the episode.

Parents will also be concerned about how to discipline their child with epilepsy. As a general rule, epileptic children should be disciplined in the same way as any other child in the family. Abnormal behaviour may be associated with a seizure but this is very much the exception rather than the rule. It would, of course, be inappropriate to discipline a child for such behaviour, as he or she has no control over it.

Adolescence is often a turbulent time for families, whether or not the adolescent family member has epilepsy. Adolescents with epilepsy will exhibit all the usual behavioural ups and downs of this period, and it is important not to relate all their behaviour to the epilepsy. However, normal adolescent behaviour can be a problem in conjunction with epilepsy. Some teenagers may reject the diagnosis of epilepsy, despite having suffered from the condition for a long time. This denial can lead to the irregular taking of medication (noncompliance), which may result in an increase in seizure frequency. In addition, adolescents tend to stay up later at night, and some experiment with alcohol and drugs. All these factors may provoke seizures. Then there is the almost universal adolescent desire to drive a car. The practicalities of this will be discussed later, but it is certainly an issue that can become contentious within a family. Often, though, it can be used to encourage compliance with medication on the basis that it is necessary to be seizure-free to obtain, and subsequently retain, a driver's licence.

OLDER PEOPLE WITH EPILEPSY

Epilepsy in the older age group is more common than in any other age group except infancy, and it is a problem that appears to be increasing with the progressive ageing of the population. For example, it is reported that there are about sixteen new cases of epilepsy per 100 000 of the population per annum in adult life, increasing to 50 new cases per 100 000 of the population over the age of 60 and up to fifteen new cases per 100 000 per annum over the age of 70.

One of the characteristics of epilepsy in this age group is that about 50 per cent or more of seizures are partial in nature. This is because strokes and other vascular events (problems relating to blood vessels), which are common among older people, produce local areas of brain damage (and subsequent partial seizures). Other characteristics of epilepsy in this age group can create diagnostic difficulties. For example, atonic seizures (previously called drop attacks), where individuals suddenly crumple to the ground, are quite common. These are often not thought to be seizures but some form of 'funny turn'. As it is frequently thought that funny turns are 'to be expected' in older people, epilepsy is frequently not diagnosed. Some form of paralysis after a seizure is also common in older people, such that a diagnosis of a transient ischaemic attack (TIA) may be made in error. In addition, there may be prolonged confusion or mild dementia for a few days after a seizure, making diagnosis difficult.

The tests used in the diagnosis of epilepsy, mainly the EEG and CT or MRI scan, are more difficult to interpret in older people, again making the diagnosis of epilepsy somewhat less certain.

As far as management is concerned, there is a general feeling that treatment with anti-epileptic medication should not be commenced unless the diagnosis is fairly sure. However, it is known that there is a high incidence of subsequent seizures after a first seizure in old age, especially if there is an underlying organic (e.g. vascular) problem. This has led to some discussion as to whether, contrary to the general rule, treatment should not, in fact, be commenced after a first seizure in older people. Having said this, the use of medications, particularly quite powerful medications such as AEDs, is not something that should be commenced lightly in the older age group. Older people are frequently taking a number of other drugs for high blood pressure, arthritis and so on, and there may be interactions between the various medications. Cognitive side effects are possible in this age group, especially with some of the older anti-epileptic drugs. In my experience, lamotrigine has been particularly useful, but needs to be introduced *very slowly*, with most patients requiring a low dosage. It has the advantage of being non sedative. Excessive dosage, as for many of the AEDs, may cause dizziness and unsteadiness, with the risk of falls. From a medical point of view, the management of epilepsy in older people is not entirely simple.

The social implications of seizures in older people should not be understated. A diagnosis of epilepsy can mean loss of independence and a tendency towards social isolation. It takes longer for older people to recover from a seizure, and they obviously require care during the recovery period. This is a serious problem if they are living on their own, and could force them into less independent living arrangements. In addition, it has been reported that there is considerable fear among older people after a seizure. The fear of having seizures in public is very real for all people with epilepsy, but it is particularly so in the older age group. It can prevent them venturing out, leaving some of them with little social contact.

The whole subject of epilepsy in old age has only just begun to receive the recognition it deserves. Hopefully, in the years to come, the time to commence treatment, appropriate medications and guidelines for overall management will become clearer than they are at present.

DISABLED PEOPLE WITH EPILEPSY

People who have sustained brain damage either from birth (cerebral palsy) or later in life may have an intellectual and/or a physical disability that can be associated with epileptic seizures. As the brain damage is permanent, the seizures are often a lifelong problem, although not necessarily difficult to control.

However, for disabled individuals with myoclonic seizures and drop attacks, control can be quite hard to achieve. It is important in this group of patients to find a suitable balance between seizure control and drug side effects. The latter are often difficult to detect, as many of the patients are unable to communicate. Drowsiness, drooling and behavioural change are quite common AED side effects in these individuals. (Drowsiness and drooling may also be part and parcel of the brain damage, however, and the medications should not always be blamed.) Behavioural problems are quite often treated with other medications that, in themselves, may compound the drowsiness and occasionally cause a deterioration in seizure control.

Many disabled epileptics are overmedicated with AEDs and sometimes with other medications such as antidepressants and tranquillisers, which may have been used to 'treat' the cognitive and behavioural side effects of the AEDs. A reduction of the medication load is often beneficial.

In this group of patients there is a need for a regular review, not only of the patients' general health, but also of their epilepsy and particularly their medications. Blood-level monitoring is often useful in an attempt to minimise drug side effects for, as mentioned, these are difficult to recognise.

Chapter 10

Pseudo-epileptic Seizures

Pseudo-epileptic seizures are episodes that superficially resemble, but are not, seizures. They are non-epileptic in origin, arising subconsciously. A number of terms, none of them perfect, are used to describe these episodes, including 'non-epileptic seizures', 'pseudo-seizures', 'psychogenic seizures' and psychic seizures'. The term 'non-epileptic attacks' is also used. In the context of this book, the term 'pseudo-epileptic seizures' (PES) will be used.

The frequency of pseudo-epileptic seizures is unclear, with estimates varying widely. However, they are seen in a specialist epilepsy setting often enough to warrant serious consideration, both medically and socially. They may occur at any stage of life, including early childhood, but are most frequent in adolescence and early adulthood. They also occur more often in women than men. They happen in individuals with or without intellectual disabilities, and in people who definitely have epilepsy as well as in those who do not.

A patient who is having a pseudo-epileptic seizure exhibits a number of features that are similar to the features of a regular seizure, but may be sufficiently different for a doctor to suspect or conclude that the seizure is not a true epileptic convulsion. Some of these features are shown in Table 10.1.

TABLE 10.1 – FEATURES THAT MAY BE HELPFUL IN DIFFERENTIATING BETWEEN CONVULSIVE PSEUDO-EPILEPTIC SEIZURES AND CONVULSIVE EPILEPTIC SEIZURES

FEATURE	EPILEPTIC SEIZURE	PSEUDO-EPILEPTIC SEIZURE
Precipitant	Usually none	Often emotional
Circumstances – in sleep – when alone	 Common Common	 Rare Less common
Onset	Usually abrupt; may be preceded by short aura	May be gradual with increasing emotional symptoms
Cry at onset	Common	Unusual
Vocalisation	During automatism	Common during seizure
Motor phenomena	Stereotyped; usually occur during both tonic and clonic phases; clonic movements slow as seizure continues	Variable; often tonic or clonic only; clonic components vary in amplitude and frequency during attack are often 'flapping' or 'thrashing; pelvic thrusting
Injury	Common	Rare
Incontinence	Common	Unusual
Tongue biting	Common	Rare
Consciousness	Usually totally lost in convulsive seizures	Variable; it is often possible to communicate with patient during attack
Restraint	No effect	Sometimes terminates attack; patient may resist
Duration of convulsion	Usually short	May be prolonged
Termination of attack	Usually short; confusion common; drowsiness or sleep common	May be gradual, often with emotional display; confusion unusual; drowsiness or sleep unusual

It is not uncommon for people with pseudo-epileptic seizures to show a progressive increase in seizure frequency despite the addition of more and more medication, or despite having tried numerous anti-epileptic drugs. In other words, the fits do not appear to respond to anything at all. While there are undoubtedly people with epilepsy whose seizures are difficult to control, ongoing seizures with ever-increasing medication should at least alert a doctor to the possibility of pseudo-epileptic seizures.

In the simplest terms, pseudo-epileptic seizures are an external manifestation of a cry for help by a troubled individual. Just as some people who are troubled or stressed develop psychological symptoms such as headache, abdominal discomfort or backache, these people develop apparent seizures or pseudo-epileptic seizures. Individuals with pseudo-epileptic seizures who do not have epilepsy may have witnessed a seizure in real life or on television, which is perhaps the reason they chose this particular set of symptoms to express their underlying troubles. Individuals who *do* have epilepsy may choose subconsciously to use their condition to manipulate or avoid situations by embellishing their symptoms from time to time. They may then progress to having pseudo-epileptic seizures in addition to genuine seizures.

In some situations, conflicts that exist within the psyche may be converted to a seizure, a process that presents an outlet for strong emotions at the same time as concealing the conflict. This conversion is called 'primary gain'. Other individuals may have pseudo-epileptic seizures in order to bring about particular reactions from other people. Some reactions may be negative, such as rejection, but they are more likely to be positive, such as the provision of more care and attention. This process is called 'secondary gain'. The achievement of secondary gain may become a prominent subconscious feature of pseudo-epileptic seizures.

Much of the literature on the subject of pseudo-epileptic seizures suggests that the outlook for people with this condition is poor. But recent studies, including observations of a substantial number of patients at Westmead Hospital in Sydney, suggest that for people who develop pseudo-epileptic seizures quite acutely and have not had them for long, the outlook for cessation of these episodes and a return to full health is excellent. For individuals who have had pseudo-epileptic seizures for a long time, often in addition to their epileptic seizures, management becomes more difficult and the chances of alleviating the condition are reduced.

Chapter 11

Epilepsy and Learning

While this chapter applies mainly to children, the relationship between epilepsy and learning is also of importance to adults, who will often wish to continue learning for much of their lives.

The future of a youngster with epilepsy depends a great deal on the management of the condition during the child's early years. The attitude adopted at home and at school is most important. Children with epilepsy need to share the company of others, go whenever possible to normal schools and partake in the usual activities. The vast majority of children with epilepsy are entirely normal from an intellectual point of view but have a particular problem – namely, epilepsy. For many children this may be less disabling, or less of an inconvenience, than a condition such as asthma or diabetes.

Some parents and teachers blame any unusual behaviour, such as temper tantrums or outbursts of anger and irritability, on the child's epilepsy. In truth, there is usually no connection between the two unless there are very good indications otherwise. However, there is evidence that in some children with epilepsy, learning problems may occur in connection with their condition.

It is reported that up to 50 per cent of boys and about 15 per cent of girls with epilepsy experience some form of learning difficulties at school. The reasons are not entirely certain, but include the following:

- *The epilepsy itself.* Only certain types of epilepsy are associated with learning difficulties. Children, especially boys, with EEG abnormalities or with focal EEG abnormalities on the left side of the brain read less well than non-epileptic children, while the reading skills of children with generalised epilepsy are similar to those of non-epileptic children.
- *The seizures themselves.* Clearly, in children with frequent seizures, particularly multiple absences during the course of the day, learning will be restricted. Hence the need to achieve the best seizure control possible.
- *The effects of anti-epileptic medications.* Some of the anti-epileptic medications, particularly the barbiturates, may affect concentration and attention span. (In adult patients there is some evidence that the long-term use of phenytoin may be associated with memory problems and possibly some intellectual deterioration. In high dosage, carbamazepine and sodium valproate may have some effect on cognitive functioning.)

Overall, it is possible that some children with epilepsy may have learning problems, and these need to be recognised and dealt with both medically and educationally. It is not uncommon for parents to have academic aspirations for their child either above or below their potential. In these cases a formal educational psychology assessment may be needed to ascertain the child's potential more accurately. Naturally, some children are less well endowed intellectually than others, irrespective of having epilepsy. Some may have other conditions besides epilepsy, or underlying brain damage for whatever reason, and therefore suffer a degree of intellectual impairment. For these children it is not likely to be their epilepsy that is the limiting factor academically, but the underlying problem.

Probably the most common problem reported by adults with epilepsy is poor memory. This appears to be more pronounced in people with complex partial seizures originating from the temporal lobe, as it is the temporal lobe that is important for memory. Ongoing uncontrolled seizures, especially if associated with taking several anti-epileptic medications, are frequently associated with significant memory problems. Improved seizure control may well be associated with some improvement in learning. Once again, from a medical point of view, it is a matter of achieving the best possible balance between seizure control and drug side effects to ensure the medications are not causing significant memory difficulties.

For a number of people with epilepsy, there is a need to accept that their condition is associated with memory problems. A simple, practical solution is to develop habits such as using lists, diaries, notepads, electronic organisers or even alarm clocks. It is interesting, however, that many people who complain of memory problems choose to do little about them. This reluctance to help themselves is their way of denying they have a problem.

As an example, a patient in her mid-thirties, who is married, has a young child and leads quite a busy life, complained a number of times of a poor memory. On one occasion she complained of a deterioration in her memory, and when asked whether she used a diary or any form of memory aid answered, 'Of course not'. When asked why not, as most people use either a diary or a notepad to remember what they have to do each day, she replied, 'If I were seen making notes, people would know I have epilepsy'. Quite simply, this woman has failed to accept her epilepsy and believes she is seen by others as being different (not normal).

Poor memory can also mean that people with epilepsy forget to take their medication. The use of a pill box that can be filled up once a week is very useful in this regard. Certainly, if people are taking several medications, the use of such a box should be almost mandatory.

Chapter 12

Epilepsy and Lifestyle

The majority of lifestyle problems can be solved with common sense, bearing in mind the following factors:

- *The severity of the seizures.* People whose seizures are often prolonged may need to remain near medical services.
- *When and how often the fits occur.* A person whose seizures occur only during sleep may have more activities open to them than someone whose seizures occur during the day. And, quite obviously, the person who has a seizure once a year is likely to approach life differently from someone who has a seizure once a week or several times a day.
- *The age of the patient.* Very young and very old patients may need supervision during certain activities.
- *Whether there are any underlying problems.* Those people who have underlying brain damage, for example, as well as seizures, will probably be restricted in their activities anyway.

When epilepsy is first diagnosed, as we have already discussed, people are often shocked and frightened. However, once the seizures are controlled and an explanation and advice are provided, their confidence will grow and they should be encouraged to lead as full a life as possible.

There are some practical guidelines that are worth mentioning here:

- *Swimming.* People with epilepsy should never swim alone. They should always inform a companion that they have epilepsy and explain what to do if a seizure occurs.
- *Scuba diving and springboard diving.* Both these activities are best avoided.
- *Bathing.* It is preferable for people with epilepsy to shower rather than to bathe, but if they wish to take a bath, they should not be left alone in the house. It would be sensible to leave the bathroom door ajar and certainly not locked. It might also be sensible to have a door that opens outwards rather than inwards, in case a seizure occurs in the bathroom where the person ends up lying on the ground, blocking an inward-opening door. It is important to make sure the bath water is reasonably shallow.
- *Showering.* If someone has a tonic clonic convulsion in the shower, it may be difficult to reach them and they might also push an arm or a leg through a glass panel. Showers should therefore be fitted with the best shatterproof glass available, or ideally with no glass at all, just a surrounding curtain. (Wire-reinforced glass is, in fact, weaker than sheet glass.) The hot tap may be turned on fully if bumped during a seizure, resulting in burns. This may be prevented by fitting a temperature-controlled device to the water system in the shower.
- *Bicycle riding.* People who do not have frequent seizures can ride a bicycle, taking the normal precautions that any other cyclist would take, including wearing a helmet.

- *Horseriding.* People with epilepsy who wish to ride a horse should wear a helmet and ride with other people.
- *Climbing.* This is not a sensible activity for people with epilepsy and should probably be avoided.
- *Cooking.* There is always concern that people with epilepsy might have a seizure while at the stove. The individual with quite frequent seizures would be wise to invest in a microwave cooker.
- *Pillows.* For those who have sleep-associated seizures, while the risk of suffocation during a seizure is very small, it does exist. Rather than a softer feather pillow, it might be best to use a safety pillow in the form of a firm foam pillow or, for young children, perhaps no pillow at all.
- *Travelling.* Epilepsy presents no constraint to travelling, but individuals who have frequent seizures need to make sensible travel arrangements. Air travel as such does not provoke seizures, but a lack of sleep on long flights and too many 'free' drinks should be avoided if possible. Travellers should always remember to take medication (or a prescription) with them, and preferably keep some of it in their hand luggage, just in case their main luggage gets lost. They should also consider obtaining a letter of explanation from their doctor about their epilepsy and the medications they are taking. Such a letter might come in useful both when dealing with customs officials in various countries and in case they have a seizure in a foreign country and need medical attention. Also, travel insurance is essential for people with epilepsy!
- *Driving.* Driving a car has become an integral part of everyday life. Not being able to drive can be inconvenient and may limit job prospects. Driving regulations vary from country to country and, in Australia, from state to state. The general rules are that individuals need to be seizure-free for one or two years, depending upon where

they live, prior to obtaining a driver's licence. In some situations – for instance, where seizures occur only during sleep – the person may be allowed to drive. The general trend worldwide is to individualise the granting of driving licences using a commonsense approach. People with epilepsy who are wishing to drive should contact their local Roads and Traffic Authority or their local epilepsy association to obtain information on the current regulations. It is important, however, for people with epilepsy to remember that driving a car is a responsibility and that restrictions are imposed for their own protection and for the protection of other road users. People who have regular seizures have a definite responsibility *not* to drive.

• *Employment.* The unpredictable nature of epilepsy means that some occupations are simply not suitable for people with the condition. When deciding on the suitability of a job, a person needs to take two factors into account: the possibility of sustaining an injury during a seizure, and the possibility of causing harm to others. What occupations, then, are not available to people with epilepsy? These vary from country to country but, in the main, the armed forces and the police force will not employ someone with epilepsy. Other proscribed occupations include piloting an aircraft, driving a public transport vehicle, operating a crane and working with heavy or dangerous machinery. Apart from these few exceptions, the vast majority of occupations and careers are open to people with epilepsy.

Chapter 13

Who is Normal?

Normality is a social judgment that varies with social trends. In addition, there is a gulf between behaviour that is legislated as being normal to avoid discrimination, and that which is actually accepted by society at large. It is suggested that normality is a variable feast and that most of us, at some time or another, might have been judged by others, or perhaps ourselves, as having behaved in an abnormal fashion.

In clinical practice, it is common to hear people with epilepsy say, 'I just want to be normal, like other people'. Although it is politically correct to say that all people with epilepsy are normal, this is not always the case, and society does not always view them as such. This relates to the personality of some individuals with epilepsy and to the nature of seizures themselves.

When we consider what some seizures look like, it is perhaps understandable that this attitude exists. Complex partial seizures, for example, sometimes involve bizarre behaviour, which may include undressing, breaking into song, making strange noises, talking nonsense, and so on. A person having a tonic clonic seizure jerks all over, possibly froths at the mouth and may be incontinent. Such a seizure may be followed by confusion and erratic behaviour, which cannot be regarded as normal behaviour in a public place. This does not mean that onlookers will not be sympathetic and helpful, but they will also be surprised, perhaps frightened, and may feel helpless.

Furthermore, the progressive closure of psychiatric and other health institutions means that more people with intellectual or physical handicaps now reside in the community. While there is little doubt that this has been a desirable move, it may also have had a negative impact on the public's perception of epilepsy. Many of these individuals have seizures as part of their underlying problem and, because society tends to generalise about things, this could lead to the misconception that all epileptics have associated handicaps. These institutional closures may have therefore coloured society's already stereotyped view of epilepsy.

So seizure-related behaviour and the association of seizures with physical/intellectual handicap make it difficult for the public to perceive people with epilepsy as being normal. This is not to suggest that the public perception is right, but people with epilepsy need to understand why such a view exists and learn how to deal with it.

In years gone by doctors used to talk of some patients with epilepsy as having 'temporal lobe personalities'. This was meant to imply that they exhibited certain personality traits such as obsessiveness, talking excessively, writing reams when a few lines would do, hyper-religious tendencies, and so on. All these traits made it difficult for them to develop friendships and maintain relationships. It is no longer acceptable to talk of a temporal lobe personality; however, some people with epilepsy, especially those with chronic, intractable seizures, often of a complex partial nature, do have personality/psychological problems that inhibit social relationships. Many of these individuals believe that all their problems are due to their epilepsy: if they became seizure-free, either with medication or perhaps surgery, then all would be well. Not only would the

99

seizures be fixed, but their lives would be revolutionised. They would have lots of friends, be able to drive, work, and so on. Sadly, this is often not so, the limitation being their personality and their ability to get on with others. This does not usually change if the seizures cease.

Research over the past two decades, looking mainly at individuals with poor seizure control and chronic epilepsy, has shown that in this group there is a higher incidence of psychosocial problems (anxiety, depression, inability to maintain relationships, unemployment, and so on) than in the general population. This may be because of the seizures themselves (their number and severity), the types of seizures (especially if they are intractable complex partial seizures), to some extent the medications, and the individual's underlying personality (irrespective of their having epilepsy).

It is important to bear in mind that all of us have moments of anxiety and depression. These are quite normal. Indeed, for people with epilepsy, a certain level of anxiety and insecurity could be viewed as a normal response to their situation:

> Life had become so good since going on to vigabatrin. Not having seizures for three months was wonderful. Life seemed almost normal and then I had one. This was one of the most depressing experiences of my life and was just like stepping back into time. Since the fit, ten days ago, I haven't been out of the house at all until coming to see you today.

This woman's pleasure in being seizure-free for some months was devastated by suddenly having a seizure, just when she was getting used to not having seizures. She felt that she had lost control of her life, she lost self-confidence, she was concerned about being left alone and she certainly believed that she could not go out on her own. It took this woman several months to get back to her usual self. Her response to the seizure, which she had not expected, was a normal response.

Seizures are often unpredictable and sudden in onset, and may occur in embarrassing or dangerous situations. By their very nature they are anxiety-provoking. Mittan (1986) has shown that fear of seizures and their consequences is widespread, although often not spoken of. As well as the seizures themselves, epileptics fear possible injury or death during a seizure, having a brain tumour or developing a mental illness. It is important that these fears, which may translate into true anxiety and even depression, be recognised and dealt with before they become established, otherwise a vicious circle may be set up. For example, an individual who is already anxious or has difficulty in relating to others may blame these difficulties on their epilepsy. This may lead to further social difficulties, more stress and, as a result, more seizures. Attention will be paid to dealing with the seizures while scant attention may be given to the underlying psychosocial problems. It may be that these are hard to alter, but the very recognition of their existence and open discussion of them and the limitations that they impose on the individual can be most helpful.

The purpose of this chapter has been to give the issue of normality a bit of an airing. Clearly there are no solutions to the problems raised, but this is not a reason for not thinking about them. Again it is important to remember that most people with epilepsy have mild epilepsy, good seizure control and lead normal lives. They are rarely recognised in or by society as having epilepsy. The problem of not appearing normal is really an issue only for those with difficult epilepsy, or for those who have associated handicaps or personality problems. These individuals require assistance in coming to grips with this added burden.

Chapter 14

Who Accepts Whom?

There are two separate but interconnected forms of acceptance relating to epilepsy: the individual's acceptance of their condition, and society's acceptance of someone who has epilepsy. Individuals who have not accepted their epilepsy are likely to have more problems in and with the general community. They often feel that they are discriminated against, or stigmatised, because of their condition. They believe that they are 'labelled' by society as having epilepsy – that people know they have epilepsy and as a result treat them differently – and this belief puts them on the defensive and makes them insecure.

First, we will look at the matter of acceptance of epilepsy by the individual, parents and the family.

It has already been suggested that at the time of diagnosis of epilepsy (and many other conditions) a grief reaction develops – grief for 'loss of health'. This takes a number of forms over time, as depicted in Figure 14.1. The stages shown will be familiar to many readers, although not everybody will go through each stage, nor will the reaction proceed at the same rate for each individual or family. Whatever the process that people go through, the ultimate objective is acceptance. Acceptance that they, or their child, have epilepsy and that this is part of their life in the same way that they might have asthma, a heart condition or any other ailment of a long-term nature.

No one wants to have epilepsy, and it is understandable that it takes a while, sometimes a very long time, for acceptance to occur. Some people, for a variety of reasons, never accept their condition, despite the problems this brings them. Lack of acceptance leaves them in variable states of anger and denial, both of which prevent them getting on with others and their lives. As a physician involved in the long-term management of people with epilepsy, I find this painful to witness.

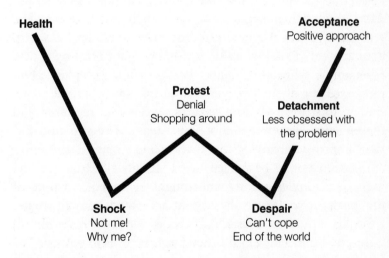

Fig. 14.1 Diagrammatic representation of the 'grief reaction', which occurs when someone dies or 'loses their health' (i.e. develops an illness such as epilepsy)

On the other hand, to witness acceptance occurring in a patient, or parent, whom one has been seeing over the years is exciting. While the acceptance sometimes results from improved seizure control, this is certainly not always the case. Something changes in the individual's or family's life that puts the epilepsy into a different perspective. It is as if it has become an inconvenience, a nuisance, rather than being the central issue or the sole topic of conversation.

This is exemplified by the case of a woman with complex partial seizures, a failed marriage and problems on moving back to the family home. Seizure control was difficult, with many seizures being stress-related. Consultations with me consisted mainly of tales of woe about the number of seizures and the limitations caused by the epilepsy, which totally dominated her life. After several years of these consultations, she arrived one day with a new hair style and began talking about the movies she had seen, dinner outings, and so on. After about ten minutes I enquired about the seizures. The reply was, 'What seizures? I am too busy and happy to worry about them!' This joyous state was brought about by a new companion, who later became her husband. Acceptance and joy lasted for about two years until marital problems arose, leading to stress and more seizures. Acceptance regressed and the epilepsy became a major issue again. The situation has since improved greatly with a divorce and a new relationship.

This example has been used specifically to put the individual's epilepsy into what might be called a 'whole of life' perspective. It also shows that acceptance may fluctuate. I would venture to suggest that this is normal. Do we not all have good and bad days; times when we feel happy or sad? Most people who have experienced the benefits of acceptance of their epilepsy, however, will not want to lose those benefits for too long, in the same way that few of us enjoy a fall in our living standards.

At this stage, the question to be asked of the reader is, 'Do you accept your epilepsy?' This does not just mean being able to say the word 'epilepsy' in public, but accepting it as part and parcel of you as an individual. If not, it might then be asked, 'Why should the general community accept you?'

This leads to the issue of acceptance of people with epilepsy in, and by, society, and the subsequent problems of discrimination, or *stigma*. Why should society not accept people with epilepsy? According to those with the condition, there are a number of possible reasons:

- *Public ignorance about epilepsy.* Studies over the years have shown this to be less of a problem than it is perceived to be by people with epilepsy, and it might be asked why the public *should* know about epilepsy. If they know about epilepsy, should they not also be informed about other chronic conditions? And how much do people with epilepsy know about diabetes, asthma, arthritis, and so on?
- *Public intolerance of people with epilepsy.* There is little evidence to support this proposal. It may be that people are frightened by seizures, but in the main they are sympathetic. Perhaps in this self-centred age the predominant feeling is one of indifference rather than intolerance. Most people would never know that a person has epilepsy, because epileptics function normally between seizures. Only when the person is having a seizure ('behaving strangely') is it recognised that they have epilepsy.
- *Public perception of an epileptic 'identity'.* Studies have certainly shown that society at large may perceive epileptics as 'nervy', highly strung, aggressive or withdrawn. There is not, however, a general view of an epileptic identity.

- *Public discrimination against people with epilepsy.* As will be argued below, this is probably more perceived than real, but the perception continues, and there is no doubt that stigma exists.

While it has been shown on numerous occasions that not all people with epilepsy feel discriminated against, or stigmatised, quite a number do. Those with a limited education, who have yet to accept their epilepsy and who have failed to gain employment, feel especially stigmatised. And there is no doubt that discrimination against people with epilepsy does occur, that stigma does exist. So what is the basis of this stigma?

Some answers to this question have come from the work of Graham Scambler (1989), who has proposed that it is conceivable that people with epilepsy threaten the social order. He has suggested several ways in which they might do this. One possibility is that epileptics are seen as dangerous, in that they are liable to sudden, unpredictable and sometimes dramatic loss of body control – they are prone to 'going berserk'. This also relates to the fear of what to do when someone has a seizure. Another possibility is that epileptics are seen as unreliable, for during their seizures they are out of control. Other views include the suggestion that because of their seizures, and their sometimes antisocial behaviour during them, epileptics are imperfect and fail to conform to culturally acceptable norms. Whichever of these views is held to be correct, readers will appreciate that there is some truth in all of them. They need to be reflected upon by everyone who deals with epilepsy, but especially by people with epilepsy who seek to understand how society sees them.

As mentioned in passing, stigma exists in two forms: real and perceived. Real stigma refers to genuine discrimination against people, solely because they have epilepsy. This excludes legitimate discrimination such as restrictions on driving a car, flying a plane, and so on. Perceived stigma is the shame felt by people with epilepsy at having the condition and the fear of being confronted by real stigma. It is the belief that people are waiting to find fault and discredit people with epilepsy because of their condition.

The difference between these two forms of stigma is very important for people with epilepsy to appreciate. The implied difference between the terms 'real' and 'perceived' does not mean that perceived stigma is any less painful. Indeed, it will be suggested that it is felt much more frequently than real stigma and is equally as painful. How it evolves is explained by the hidden distress model (Scambler & Hopkins, 1989), which follows:

1. When a diagnosis of epilepsy is made, the individual or family rapidly comes to see being an epileptic as a social liability. They adopt a 'special view of the world', which is dominated by a fear of being stigmatised (real stigma).
2. This special view of the world encourages them to hide their condition so that others will see them as being normal. They develop a policy of not declaring their epilepsy.
3. The policy of hiding their epilepsy reduces the opportunities for others to stigmatise them. But like some of the anti-epileptic drugs, it has side effects. It leads to the development of perceived stigma and the ongoing fear of real stigma. This disrupts people's lives more than would the occasional bout of real stigma.

In other words, while real stigma may occur from time to time, it is likely to be quite infrequent, although distressing. Concealment leads to ongoing perceived stigma, which may become a way of life, with unremitting pain and anguish.

Patrick West (1986) looked at the question of concealment in families who have a child with epilepsy. His observations are applicable, however, to people of all ages with epilepsy. The main dilemma seems to be whether or not to disclose the epilepsy. Where seizures occur unpredictably and are associated with antisocial behaviour, concealing the condition often seems to people to be a good idea. However, hiding the epilepsy leads to the risk of misadventure – what happens if the person has a seizure in the company of people who have no idea that the person has epilepsy? Disclosing the condition means that others are at least forewarned, and can diminish some of the risks associated with seizures.

West identified three main patterns of behaviour with regard to concealment:

- *Successful concealment.* Where the person or family makes sure that the epilepsy remains unknown to almost everyone.
- *Failed concealment.* Where the person or family remains committed to concealment, despite the fact that the epilepsy has been discovered, usually because the epileptic has been seen to have a seizure.
- *Disclosure.* Where the person or family is open about the epilepsy from the start, or the attempts to conceal the problem have failed.

The outcome of these patterns of behaviour is summarised in Table 14.1. In essence, people who successfully conceal their epilepsy continue to feel perceived stigma, as the reactions of those around them are never tested. (In the main, when they are tested, they are not what was expected. Reactions are usually positive, and this encourages the individual to look at changing their views.) Successful concealment implies social isolation with little activity outside the home. Failed concealers are drop-outs of the school of successful concealers. In simple terms, their cover has been blown. Their reaction to their failure is to work even harder at concealing their epilepsy, making the concealment almost a way of life, which causes even more problems. Only the disclosers live normal lives, reinforcing the need for disclosure, if at all possible.

While it is difficult to assess the extent of real stigma, all the evidence suggests that perceived stigma is a much greater problem. If an individual is to have the power to deal with the problem they must: first, recognise that it exists; secondly, come to accept their epilepsy; and finally, feel motivated to do something about it. The longer the stigma has been perceived, the longer it is likely to take to correct. As the reader will appreciate, acceptance and stigma are closely linked, and for those people who never come to accept their epilepsy, the stigma persists.

TABLE 14.1 – PATTERNS OF CONCEALMENT

STIGMA STRATEGY		COROLLARY		OUTCOME IN FAMILY
Successful concealing	+	Avoidance of outside activity	→	Overprotection 'Fragile child'
Failed concealing	+	Avoidance of outside activity	→	Rejection 'Defective child' (A)
		↑ ↓		
		Stigmatisation		
Disclosure	+	Participation in outside activity	→	'Normal' (B)

(A) Essentially, the child is seen as defective because of the epilepsy.

(B) As normal as can be expected, taking into account the natural parental response to the diagnosis of epilepsy.

It is common for all of us to have a down day. For someone with a chronic condition such as epilepsy, a regular down day is often explained by their epilepsy. 'If I did not have epilepsy, this would not have happened to me.' They may feel temporarily stigmatised by whatever has depressed them. I would suggest that this is normal, and sporadic episodes such as this should not be a cause for concern.

The final word on this issue is left to Catherine, a journalist with epilepsy, who describes her epilepsy and her experiences with concealment, disclosure and acceptance. 'Learning to Live With It' is her story:

At 9 am on 31 October, 1980 – half an hour before I was to sit the biology paper in my Higher School Certificate – my life took an interesting turn. I collapsed in the classroom, lost consciousness and was spirited away in an ambulance. I didn't know it then, but I had just experienced my first seizure.

Peering into the back of the ambulance, the local doctor examined me and then informed my shell-shocked mother I was suffering nervous exhaustion and needed immediate bed rest. She dutifully complied; I never sat the exam, and five weeks later, in the early hours of the morning, I had my second seizure.

I was promptly referred to a neurologist in Sydney, where the results of a lumbar puncture, EEG and CAT scan revealed I had idiopathic epilepsy. Encouragingly, I was told I did not have meningitis, I did not have encephalitis, I did not have a brain tumour and I was not going to die. While the doctor could not establish a cause for the epilepsy, he concluded it was probably genetic on my father's side.

My parents heaved a collective sigh of relief and I wondered if I would ever learn to spell 'carbamazepine', let alone pronounce it. As I sat bobbing and weaving in the chair, I also wondered how much longer I could hold on before I threw up in the doctor's surgery, thanks to the dye that had been injected into my veins during the CAT scan. Quickly my father shook the doctor's hand, my mother paid the bill and we made a hasty retreat.

I decided to defer my place at university in 1981 and, in retrospect, that was a good thing. The first six months of the year were rough, largely because my body was less than impressed with the effects of my anticonvulsant. I slept fourteen hours a day, but still managed to feel tired. I gained some weight, but ate no more than usual. I was vague, irascible and often depressed. But above all else, I was ashamed. Why, of all the diseases on this planet, did I have to be saddled with epilepsy? Forevermore, I could see myself being discussed as 'that girl with the mental deficiency, you know, the one with the kangaroos loose in the top paddock'. My friends were meeting new people and kicking up their heels at university and here was I, stuck at home in the country with my parents, learning to live with a disease I didn't want and begrudgingly swallowing pills morning and night.

I cornered the market in self-pity, although I was the last to admit it. My moods swung like the proverbial pendulum. Mum and Dad deserved a VC for putting up with me. Anyone who knows children knows a seventeen-year-old daughter is punishment enough. Now they had to contend with a seventeen-year-old daughter with epilepsy. A decoration for bravery was the least they should have expected. As far as I was concerned, though, I had every right to behave as if my life was over. Good God, epilepsy! Why didn't my neurologist just shoot me and be done with it?

As the year progressed, and my body adjusted to its daily shot of Tegretol, my health improved and, thankfully, so did my behaviour. In spite of this, I refused point-blank to tell anyone – except my immediate family – that I was epileptic. In fact, I made every effort to blowtorch the word from my vocabulary. I concluded the best way to deal with my condition was to ignore it.

111

After all, I reasoned, the general community had a pretty dim view of the disease, so why should I subject myself to prejudicial treatment unnecessarily? My strategy was simple: if I wanted to live a normal life, I had to carry on as if nothing had happened.

The following year I started at the University of New South Wales in Sydney. Understandably, Mum was frantic about this move away from home. Up till now she had been the one who reminded me every day it was time to take my tablets. Too often, though, it wasn't just a reminder, it was a plea. When I was feeling low I would stupidly, but steadfastly, refuse to take my medication, knowing full well the implications of such a pig-headed act. I hated taking those damn tablets and I offered every irrational excuse known to man to avoid the ritual. She would gently persist and I would invariably burst into tears, sobbing at the injustice of it all. From now on, we both knew the onus of responsibility lay with me. Given my track record, Mum had every reason to view this prospect with great trepidation.

My charade began in earnest even before the academic year commenced. I needed a medical certificate to accompany my application to one of the university's residential colleges. I spoke to our family doctor, who was happy to supply one. Quite correctly, he indicated that I suffered from idiopathic epilepsy, had had two seizures, but was well controlled on 600 milligrams of Tegretol daily. He added that, apart from the epilepsy, my general health was excellent.

I was horrified. What the hell was this man thinking about? Didn't he appreciate the enormous social stigma attached to epilepsy? I doubled back to get a new certificate, determined all references to my epilepsy be expunged. In tears, I told him if the warden of the college found out I had epilepsy, I may as well set fire to my application before I sent it. Indeed, I would be left without a roof over my head and I could kiss university goodbye.

The doctor tried to reassure me that, far from wanting to weed me out as some monster from the Black Lagoon, the college simply wanted to know if I might require special attention in a medical emergency. It was standard procedure. Sure, and Hitler was a saint, too! The words of my GP fell on deaf ears and I was damned if I would take the risk. I became increasingly agitated. After all, I was the one who had something wrong with her brain. Who better to know about the public's prejudice toward people with a dysfunctional brain than the victim herself? As far as I was concerned, I had no reason to assume the attitude of the college warden would be any different – and I was not about to give him the benefit of the doubt. It was a new medical certificate or *nothing*.

Badgered into submission and obviously feeling sorry for this teary creature in front of him, he reluctantly agreed to my request. He stressed, however, that I could not keep my epilepsy a secret forever. Holding the new certificate close to me, I walked from his rooms and mumbled to myself triumphantly, 'You wanna bet?'

For the next two years I worked overtime to make sure no one got wind of my affliction. I made sure my tablets were always hidden from view. Much to Mum's consternation, I chose not to wear a medical bracelet for fear my fellow students caught sight of it at mealtimes or during lectures.

If I went to the local watering hole with friends, I was always quizzed about why I drank so little. Not surprisingly, there was an exponential relationship between the amount of liquor they consumed and the amount of flak I copped for being too sober too often. They noticed I only ever had one beer or one glass of wine before I moved on to the lime and sodas. In fact, no one had ever seen me drunk. What was my problem? My sobriety became a running joke and people soon tired of my excuses. Antibiotics. The flu. Had to study for an exam. Sister was visiting the next morning. You name it, I invented it. Not once, however, did I offer them the truth: that if I mixed too much alcohol with my anticonvulsant, I ran the risk of inducing a seizure.

Any appointment I had with my neurologist became a check-up at the dentist or a trip to the movies or a visit to see relatives. I came to dread those appointments like the plague because they meant I had to have an EEG, and that, of course, meant my head had to be fitted with electrodes and plastered with a revolting, gooey chemical, which helped the equipment read the electrical discharges in my brain. This was not painful, but it was embarrassing. Not only did I have to ride home on the bus with parts of the stubborn residue still glued to my head, but I also had to hope desperately no one would see me as I bolted back to my college room and into the shower.

On one occasion I didn't make it. A couple of male students standing in the corridor wanted to know what I'd done to my hair. Although I was sure I sounded convincing, somehow there was something not quite right about a three-year-old vigorously shaking a can of cola and opening it in front of my head. A height difference of more than half a metre for starters! It was a ridiculous story and their incredulous expressions confirmed as much.

By the end of 1993, however, I was feeling pretty smug. Three years had passed since the diagnosis of epilepsy had been made, and no one at uni was any the wiser. For all intents and purposes, I was as normal as the next person. I was happily ensconced in college life and had made some great friends. One of these was Tess, a dairy farmer's daughter from Bodalla in New South Wales. She was a straight-talking, no-nonsense country girl with a brilliant sense of humour and we got on like a house on fire. It also happened we had similar interests, and one of these was to spend part of our summer vacation backpacking around New Zealand.

There was little scope for manoeuvre in our tight itinerary. We planned to cover the country from top to bottom in four weeks. There were a lot of late nights and a lot of early mornings and a lot of long days travelling. The 13 kilograms I carried on my back guaranteed I was dog-tired at the end of every day. As the trip became more interesting, I became less diligent about taking my medication, but still I felt fine. Our final night saw us bed down early at a youth hostel in Auckland. Sadly, we would be on our way back to Sydney at 9.30 am the next day after a sensational holiday. Tess didn't know it, but I had one thing left to do before we left New Zealand, and that was to have a severe generalised seizure in the bunk next to her three hours before our departure.

Groggy, dazed and sore, I regained consciousness in the Accident and Emergency ward of Auckland Hospital. I had no idea what day it was, what time it was or how I had come to be there. A young registrar was standing over me checking my pupils with his ophthalmoscope. When I asked him what had happened, he told me that Tess and the hostel warden had brought me in after I suffered what appeared to be a prolonged seizure as I awoke from sleep. He gently reassured me that everything was all right, explained I would be a bit confused for a few hours and said I was lucky to have a supportive friend who understood my condition. I looked up at him and said, 'Actually, she doesn't. I never told her.' Those words cut dead our amicable exchange instantly. His stinging rebuke, so unexpected, made me flinch. 'How dare you travel to another country with someone you call a friend and not tell her you have epilepsy? Do you have rocks in your head, woman?' The tears started to roll down my cheeks, but they cut no ice with the angry young man in front of me. 'Get off that bed now and get out there and apologise to that poor girl. I don't care how sick you feel; you owe her that much.' He shook his head and marched out of the room. To say I had made a bloody fine mess of everything was a masterpiece of understatement.

Tess jumped to her feet as I swayed into the waiting area. By this time the registrar had spoken to her. She steadied me with her hand and we both sat down. The look of relief on her face was unmistakable, but so, too, was the hurt. 'Why, Cath? Why didn't you tell me? I had no idea. I thought you were dying and I didn't know how to help you. You scared the living daylights out of me! If only you'd told me I could have reminded you to take your tablets. Made sure you got more sleep. Anything!'

That was the cue. I cried, she cried, and in between my sobs all I could say was 'I'm sorry'. In all my life I don't think I've ever felt as lousy as I felt that day. For three years I'd kept my secret, but at what cost? I'd jeopardised one of my most valued friendships; I'd deceived a lot of people who cared about me; I'd convinced myself I was a social outcast and conveniently blamed society for it. I had failed to share with others the wealth of information I'd gathered about epilepsy and, most importantly, I'd been dishonest with myself by not accepting the truth: I was an epileptic, I would always be an epileptic and nothing on God's earth was going to change that.

It was a bruising life lesson, but one for which I will be eternally grateful. Miraculously, we caught our plane (only because our 110-kilo Maori taxi driver broke the land speed record to get us to the airport), and I returned to Australia a different person. Realistically, I knew I would always be disappointed that I had epilepsy, but I now knew I wouldn't be ashamed of it or try to hide it like I had before. I decided that if people ostracised me on the grounds of my having a chemical abnormality in the brain, it was my good fortune because they were bigger morons than me and I didn't want to know them anyway.

And, of course, people didn't reject me. Come to think of it, they didn't even sprint to the other side of the street when they saw me coming. They did what any normal, inquisitive, caring human being would do and that was ask questions. They wanted to know what caused epilepsy, what it was like to have a seizure, whether the seizures hurt me, how I prevented them, whether I took medication, whether there was anything I couldn't do because I had epilepsy. The list went on and on. But, over-whelmingly, the two most asked questions were: how do we recognise a seizure and how do we help you if you have one? People genuinely cared. I was astonished, but I shouldn't have been because these were the self-same questions I would have asked if the boot was on the other foot. I'd been so caught up with my desperate struggle to appear 'normal', I'd overlooked the fact that none of us really are. I happened to draw epilepsy in the genetic lottery, but I could quite easily have pulled out diabetes or asthma or cystic fibrosis or spina bifida or multiple sclerosis or a million other disorders I don't have the space, time or inclination to mention.

In the ten years since that New Zealand registrar wiped the floor with me, I've talked openly and honestly about my epilepsy with anyone who's willing to listen. Sometimes I'm sure they haven't been willing, but I've bored them witless with the facts and figures anyway. I came to the conclusion a long time ago that if I didn't do everything in my power to educate the non-epileptics around me, I was not only being derelict in my duty, I also stood the very real risk of having 1600 dollars of good dental work renovated by some well-meaning maniac with a spoon! In fact, if I had a dollar for every time I've calmly squealed, *'Epileptics do not swallow their tongue'*, I wouldn't be sitting here writing this story now; I'd be cruising the Caribbean on my luxury yacht.

In spite of my condition, I think I've achieved quite a bit. I graduated from university. I have a driver's licence. I've worked happily as a journalist for the best part of eight years, both in Australia and overseas. I've travelled extensively. I've met many remarkable people and made lifelong friends in the process. What's more, I've publicly acknowledged my epilepsy and learnt to live with it. Sure, I'm one of the lucky ones. I take only one anticonvulsant medication, I'm well controlled and my seizures, though rare, occur in the early morning while I'm in bed. This notwithstanding, I still live with a time bomb and I treat it with the respect it deserves. I haven't missed a tablet in over five years;

I get lots of sleep and drink very little; I exercise religiously to help me cope with the chronic tiredness I suffer at the hands of my medication, and I make no apology to anyone for living my life this way.

For many epileptics, though, this is not the case. They guard their secret with their life and live in fear that others will find out. I knew one such man. While working in London I responded to an advertisement in the 'Share Accommodation' pages of *The Times* newspaper. Cathy was looking for three other people to move into her West Kensington flat. After countless interviews she decided Gill the Scot, Owen the Irishman and me the ring-in from another hemisphere were the perfect combination to promote international goodwill and, hopefully, do the dishes on a regular basis. We decided dinner at a good restaurant was the best way to get to know each other. During the meal I told my flatmates I had epilepsy. They were terribly sympathetic, asked what to do if I had a seizure and told me they were grateful I had been honest with them. Gill then went to the bathroom, Cathy went to the bar and Owen leaned over to me and whispered, 'Just between you and me and the wall, I've got epilepsy, too!'

'So why the hell are you telling me this great tale in their absence?' I roared. 'Shhhh,' he pleaded. 'I will not shhhh, you idiot. You know you have an obligation to tell Cathy and Gill exactly what you've just told me.' I realised later my memory was very short. The two girls walked back to the table, our conversation stopped dead and I flashed Owen a look that would have scorched the soles off his shoes. The poor guy sat there motionless. He said nothing then, but as the night wore on I think a little bit of guilt and a lot of pleasant wine provided the impetus for him to do the right thing. He was deeply self-conscious and embarrassed as he discussed his epilepsy – I don't think the man had ever talked openly about it before in his life, and he was thirty years of age. Far from being judgmental or critical, Cathy and Gill were more interested in the bizarre statistics. Wow! In a city of ten million people, what was the probability of getting *two* epileptics together in the *same* household?

Unfortunately, that was the last time Owen talked about his condition. He made it very clear the subject was now closed. Several weeks later he had quite a serious generalised seizure coming out of sleep. Cathy flapped around him like a mother hen. She changed his sheets, washed his clothes, made him a cup of tea, rang his work to say he was sick and did everything she could to make him comfortable. All she got for her trouble was a mouthful of abuse when she picked up the phone to call an ambulance. You see, Owen was a doctor studying to be a neurologist, and he would have cut off his right leg before he allowed himself to be admitted to a casualty ward with an epileptic attack. It was suddenly abundantly clear: if you were a neurological specialist, you diagnosed the disease, you didn't suffer with it.

Well, Owen was very wrong. Epilepsy belongs to all of us, either directly or indirectly, and for my money I'd rather face it than fear any day.

It would be difficult to say anything more after these candid comments!

Chapter 15

To Declare or
Not to Declare?

The question of disclosure, for which there is no universal answer, remains a difficult one for people with epilepsy.

The general advice must be to encourage people with epilepsy to declare their condition. However, this should be done in an informed way once they understand their epilepsy so that they can say more than just 'I have epilepsy'. Their declaration is their educational contribution to the community and will go at least some way to decreasing the stigma, real or perceived, that surrounds epilepsy.

Nevertheless, it takes some people considerable courage to declare their epilepsy, especially those who have very occasional seizures or seizures only arising from sleep. They may feel that it is unnecessary to declare their condition, depending, of course, on the circumstances in which they find themselves. If not telling someone about their epilepsy places the other person in a difficult or dangerous situation, however infrequent the seizures might be, this is unfair.

Some people hide their epilepsy because they themselves have not come to grips with it. They feel controlled and defeated by their epilepsy and do not wish to discuss it. After years of clinical practice in the field of epilepsy, it has become apparent to me that however many times some people are advised to declare their epilepsy, they will not do so. Of course, that is their prerogative, but having seizures means the individual has some degree of responsibility to others, particularly with regard to driving. For this reason, it is very important that people with ongoing seizures make their condition known both to their doctor and to the Roads and Traffic Authority. It is essentially negligent on their part not to do so.

People may also conceal their condition in order to remain in a line of work that might not be regarded as suitable for people with epilepsy. This is exemplified by the case of a man (Mr A.), in his mid-thirties, who had been working in the 'rag trade' for many years as a cutter. He was good at his job and, while he had occasional daytime tonic clonic seizures, most of his fits occurred in the evenings or early mornings. He had never declared his epilepsy to his employers on the basis they might perceive him as being 'abnormal', to use his own expression.

Part of his job involved cutting material using an electronically operated blade. Although it had a guard, it was not entirely safe if someone were to fall onto it. The inevitable happened. He had a seizure at work and fell onto the blade, but fortunately was not injured. His employer was terrified when called to the scene, feeling considerable concern for his employee for whom he had a high regard and who had been in his employ for some years. Out of concern, he suggested to Mr A. that he shift to another part of the business rather than be exposed to this particular danger. This was interpreted by Mr A. as implying that he wasn't good enough for the job because he had epilepsy. Despite numerous explanations, a meeting between Mr A., the employer and a member of the clinic staff, and a visit to the cutting room, Mr A. could not be dissuaded from believing he was being discriminated against because of his epilepsy. He resigned and found similar work at another establishment where, again, he chose not to inform his employers of his epilepsy. It might be worth mentioning that this same man was also driving without having declared his epilepsy. As a result, his driver's licence was withdrawn for a time until he came to grips with the social responsibility that his seizures imposed upon him. From a physician's point of view, dealing with these sorts of problems can be frustrating, especially when all attempts at logic fail.

The question of declaring or not declaring one's epilepsy remains a vexed and difficult one, but cannot be ignored. It is important to discuss this problem with family, close friends, your doctor or any other person with whom you feel you can talk openly. You need a sounding board to try to think through this undoubtedly problematic issue. For those of us who are involved in the management of epilepsy, it is very easy to say, 'Yes, you should declare your epilepsy', but equally we need to recognise that, under certain circumstances, this may be very hard to do.

Chapter 16

Having Control over Your Epilepsy

As will have become apparent in the preceding chapters, when talking about epilepsy there are two forms of control: seizure control, and the individual's feeling of control (or lack of it) over their epilepsy.

Individuals with frequent seizures may well feel that their epilepsy dominates their lives and that they have little control over it. However, it is not uncommon for some individuals with quite infrequent seizures to react the same way. They may go weeks or months without a seizure, yet still feel loss of control and self-confidence when one occurs, possibly reflecting their underlying personality traits. Other people are remarkable in that, despite their very frequent seizures – perhaps they have several a day – they nevertheless manage to work and lead full lives with the exception of driving. One wonders what these people might have achieved without their epilepsy, although it may well be the epilepsy itself that has strengthened their resolve and prompted them to make the very best of their lives.

There can, however, be little doubt that epileptics who come to grips with their epilepsy, who accept it as part and parcel of their lives and who regard it predominantly as an inconvenience, feel they have control over their lives – most of the time. It is unusual for people to feel in control of their epilepsy all of the time, just as very few of us feel in control of our lives and everything around us all the time. It is certainly a major achievement when, for the most part, they establish this feeling of control.

Being well informed about your epilepsy, your medications and the implications for the future, as well as being prepared to openly discuss your epilepsy, are all manifestations of acceptance. Acceptance implies having control over your epilepsy and your life.

Epilogue

Looking to the Future

This book is somewhat different from the preceding ones I have written, reflecting my growing feeling that the social aspects and implications of epilepsy are just as important as the medical aspects. I hope to have been forthright in tackling what might be seen as contentious issues – questions of normality, acceptance, stigma and declaring one's epilepsy – about which a degree of political correctness is usually expected. It is not suggested the views presented here are necessarily correct. They merely represent a distillation of my experience gained over the past two decades of listening to epileptics, the parents of epileptic children and carers. They are not designed to provide answers but rather to provoke individuals to think about these matters in a socially responsible way. Naturally, some people will disagree strongly with some of the views expressed. That is normal and healthy.

Overwhelmingly, though, the message of this book is one of hope. The outlook for people with epilepsy in the new millennium is definitely very much better than it was ten years ago. A better understanding of the basic mechanisms of epilepsy, much greater interest amongst health professionals in epilepsy, the advent of new drugs, improved surgical techniques and the growing recognition that the social aspects associated with epilepsy are important, all bode well for the future. Sadly, this does not mean that some individuals with difficult, or ill-controlled, epilepsy will not continue to have problems. However, it is likely that the numbers of people with ill-controlled epilepsy will decrease over time and the quality of life for the majority of people with epilepsy will continue to improve.

Epilepsy education, especially for those with epilepsy and for their families, as well as for the general community, needs to gather momentum. People with epilepsy must be the catalysts for change. It is they who must tackle the stigma, real or perceived. Only when they are well informed about their own epilepsy and have accepted it will they be able to do this.

There *is* hope for the future, for those who grasp it. As Charles Birch wrote in *Regaining Compassion for Humanity and Nature*:

Hope is not the superficial by-product of favourable circumstances; it springs from one's character, from what one is and cares about, and believes in. The seventeenth century poet John Gay wrote, 'While there is life there is hope'. A deeper truth emerges when this saying is reversed, 'Where there is hope there is life'.

Appendix 1

Medications Used in the Treatment of Epilepsy

DRUGS CURRENTLY USED

Any side effects related to excessive (over) dosage are in *italics*.

Carbamazepine

Carbamazepine is available as 100 mg and 200 mg tablets, 200 mg and 400 mg slow-release tablets and a suspension (100 mg/5 ml).

Side effects with carbamazepine are few but include sleepiness and *double vision*; these symptoms usually mean that the patient is taking too much medicine. A rash like measles may occur during the first month of treatment. If it does, the patient is sensitive to the drug and should probably stop taking it after discussion with their doctor.

Patients on carbamazepine should avoid taking the antibiotic erythromycin, as it may make the blood level of carbamazepine rise and produce toxicity. The same applies to the heart drug Verapamil, and the anti-ulcer medication cimetidine. Carbamazepine also renders the oral contraceptive pill less effective, so a high-dose or alternative form of contraception may be required.

Clobazam

Clobazam is available as a 10 mg tablet. It is not a drug that is often used on its own; it needs to be used with another anticonvulsant (adjunct therapy). It can be taken once or twice daily. Side effects are few, but include some drowsiness, weight gain and, occasionally, depression. Tolerance may occur (that is, the patient 'gets used' to the drug).

Clonazepam

Clonazepam is available in 0.5 mg and 2.0 mg tablets and as a liquid (2.5 mg/ml). Clonazepam generally needs to be taken two or three times a day. Side effects are quite frequent, more so in children than adults. They include hyperactivity, weight increase, drowsiness, *slurred speech* and an *unsteady walk* (as if drunk). There may also be increased salivation. As with clobazam, in some patients, tolerance occurs. In these patients, seizures may recur, usually one to six months after treatment was begun.

Ethosuximide

Ethosuximide is available as a 250 mg capsule and a syrup (250 mg/5 ml). It lasts a long time in the body and so may be taken once a day, although it is usually given twice daily. Side effects are few and include a decrease in appetite, abdominal pain, tiredness, headache and an unsteady walk.

Gabapentin

Gabapentin is available as a 100 mg, 300 mg and 400 mg capsule, and a 600 mg and 800 mg tablet. Ideally, it should be taken three times a day and quite often in high dosage. It is of help largely in partial seizures and can occasionally make absences and myoclonus worse. Side effects include weight gain and drowsiness.

Lamotrigine

This AED is available as 5 mg, 25 mg, 50 mg, 100 mg and 200 mg tablets. It has been shown to be effective in both partial and generalised seizures. It is helpful in the Lennox-Gastaut Syndrome, difficult absence seizures and atonic seizures. Lamotrigine needs to be introduced slowly, especially in people also taking sodium valproate. Side effects include a rash (mainly in association with sodium valproate), insomnia (rarely) and, when taken with carbamazepine, sometimes double vision and an unsteady walk.

Levetiracetam

This AED should become available in Australia by the middle of 2003 as 250 mg, 500 mg and 1000 mg tablets. It is useful in partial seizure disorders and is taken twice daily. The main side effects are tiredness, headache and drowsiness.

Nitrazepam

Nitrazepam is available as a 5 mg tablet and is given once or twice daily. Side effects are similar to those described for clonazepam, but to a much lesser extent.

Oxcarbazepine

This AED is a modification of carbamazepine, with more theoretical than actual advantages. It is available as a 150 mg and 300 mg tablet. The side effect profile is similar to that of carbamazepine.

Phenobarbitone

Phenobarbitone is available as a 30 mg tablet; for infants, pharmacists will make up a suspension, usually 15 mg/5 ml. Phenobarbitone lasts a long time in the body and can be given once daily, although it is usually given twice a day.

It has been used for many years as an anticonvulsant, but tends to make patients rather drowsy. Children and older people may behave the opposite way and become hyperactive. These behavioural changes have made phenobarbitone less popular than it used to be.

Patients on phenobarbitone should not take warfarin (to thin the blood), phenylbutazone (for arthritis), prednisone (for arthritis or asthma) or doxycycline (for infections) without careful medical supervision. Phenobarbitone also reduces the efficacy of the oral contraceptive pill.

Phenytoin

Phenytoin is available in 30 mg capsules, 50 mg tablets (chewable), 100 mg capsules and two suspensions (30 mg/ 5 ml and 100 mg/5 ml). Phenytoin is retained in the body for a long time and can be used once daily. It is available for intravenous use in emergency situations, but it can cause problems in the vein into which it is injected or in the tissues locally. A newer modification of phenytoin, fosphenytoin, is available and is less troublesome in this regard.

Phenytoin has rather a lot of side effects, although many patients' seizures are well controlled on this drug with minimal side effects. *Drowsiness*, *double vision*, an *unsteady walk* and *slurred speech* suggest that the patient is taking too much of the drug and should contact their doctor. Other side effects include swelling of the gums, rashes, acne and an increase in body hair.

Patients on phenytoin should not take rifampicin (for tuberculosis), chloramphenicol (for infections), phenylbutazone (for arthritis), dicoumarol (to thin the blood) or cimetidine (for stomach ulcers) without careful medical supervision. Phenytoin also reduces the efficacy of the oral contraceptive pill.

Primidone

Primidone is available as a 250 mg tablet. The drug is broken down to phenobarbitone in the body. (See Phenobarbitone.)

Sodium Valproate

Sodium valproate is available as a 100 mg crushable tablet, a 200 mg and 500 mg enteric-coated tablet, a syrup (200 mg/ 5 ml) and a sugar-free liquid (200 mg/5 ml). Sodium valproate stays in the body for quite a long time and may be given once daily. It is more usual to give it twice daily.

The side effects of sodium valproate are relatively few and include drowsiness, an increase in weight, hair loss (which is usually temporary) and, very rarely, jaundice (turning yellow). This last complication is serious and requires immediate medical attention. It occurs very rarely and is due to liver damage caused by the drug. If a patient taking this medication feels generally unwell, unduly tired or drowsy and has an increase in seizure frequency, a doctor should be consulted immediately.

Sulthiame

This AED, which is available as a 50 mg and 200 mg tablet, is of use in most seizure types and also has a reputation for having calming effects on behaviour. The main side effects include drowsiness, tingling of the hands and feet, loss of appetite and occasionally insomnia. When used with phenytoin it may increase phenytoin blood levels, leading to toxicity; and when used with sodium valproate, it quite often causes significant drowsiness.

Tiagabine

Available as 5 mg, 10 mg and 15 mg tablets, this medication should be taken three times a day. It is useful in treating partial seizures. The predominant side effects are dizziness, drowsiness, word-finding problems and mood changes. It has occasionally been reported to cause non-convulsive *status epilepticus*.

Topiramate

This medication is available as 25 mg, 50 mg, 100 mg and 200 mg tablets, and 15 mg, 25 mg and 50 mg sprinkle capsules. Topiramate is useful in partial seizures, to some extent in the primary generalised epilepsies, and may be of help in infantile spasms and the Lennox-Gastaut Syndrome. It interacts with carbamazepine, phenytoin and phenobarbitone, reducing the blood levels of these agents. Side effects are quite frequent and include loss of appetite, weight loss, tingling of the hands and feet, clouding of thinking, word-finding problems, mood changes, a 1 per cent chance of kidney stones and, rarely, the possible development of glaucoma. These side effects should not discourage the use of topiramate, but patients should know what to look out for.

Vigabatrin

Vigabatrin is available as 500 mg tablets and 500 mg sachets. The dose is usually taken twice a day. Side effects include drowsiness and, rarely, behavioural disturbance, especially in people with previous psychological/psychiatric problems. There are no significant interactions between vigabatrin and other medications. Over the last few years, 10–30 per cent of people taking vigabatrin on a long-term basis are reported to have developed a loss of peripheral vision. This seems to occur in two forms of severity: the minority of people are symptomatic, they cannot see out at the periphery and bump into things, or drop things they reach out for; others have visual field loss on formal eye testing, but are asymptomatic.

The loss seems to be permanent even if the medication is ceased. This side effect has greatly reduced the use of vigabatrin; however, it is still used in the treatment of infantile spasms and may be appropriate in some people with partial seizures if other medications have failed, provided the person is made fully aware of the risks.

The following table summarises the effectiveness of the various AEDS relative to different seizure types, provides information on the usefulness of blood-level monitoring and lists the common side effects of each medication.

ANTI-EPILEPTIC DRUGS (AED)
EFFICACY IN PARTICULAR TYPES OF EPILEPSY, AND IMPORTANT SIDE EFFECTS

AED (TRADE NAME)		PARTIAL SEIZURES†	PRIMARY GENERALISED EPILEPSY	WESTS/ LENNOX-GASTAUT	SIDE EFFECTS (AND OTHER ISSUES)
Barbiturates	*	+	++	+	Behavioural problems in children, sedation. Memory deterioration and general functional slowing with long-term use
Dilantin	***	++	+	+	Gum swelling, acne, increased body hair, hard to individualise dosage and needs, regular blood tests
Epilim	*	++	++++	++	Weight gain, hair loss, liver damage (very rare), risk of polycystic ovaries, risk of foetal abnormalities
Frisium	*	++	++	++	Weight gain, drowsiness, behaviour change (tolerance may occur = effect wears off)
Gabitril	*	+	–	–	Dizziness, drowsiness, mood changes
Keppra	*	++	?	?	Headache, drowsiness
Lamictal	*	+++	+++	++	Dizzy, double vision, insomnia, rash (avoidable with slow introduction)
Mogadon	*	–	+	++	Irritability, drooling (children)
Neurontin	*	+	Absences w Myoclonus w	–	Weight gain, drowsiness (needs to be taken three times a day in quite high dosages)

Drug	Usefulness of blood level monitoring				Side effects
Ospolot	*	?	++	++	Drowsiness, insomnia, pins and needles of hands and feet
Rivotril	*	++	++	+	Drowsiness, irritability, withdrawal seizures on cessation, drooling (children)
Sabril	*	–	Absences w Myoclonus w	+++	Loss of peripheral vision (which may be permanent), weight gain, mood change
Tegretol	**	–	Absences w Myoclonus w	+++	Dizzy, double vision, drowsiness, rash (avoidable with slow introduction)
Topamax	*	+	+	+++	Loss of appetite, weight loss, tingling of hands/ feet, 1% risk of kidney stones. Dose-dependent: unclear thinking, problems with word-finding, glaucoma
Trileptal	*	–	Absences w Myoclonus w	+++	As for Tegretol
Zarontin	*	–	Absences only	–	Headache, nausea, abdominal discomfort

Usefulness of blood level monitoring:

***	=	useful
**	=	occasionally useful
*	=	little or no use

w = may get worse

†Partial seizures with or without secondarily generalised convulsion.

Side effects: Remember that many people will get few, or no side effects, but you still need to know what they are.

Effectiveness of AED:

++++	=	highly effective
+++	=	very effective
++	=	quite effective
+	=	little effect
–	=	no effect
?	=	uncertain effect

Appendix 2

TRADE NAMES OF COMMONLY USED ANTICONVULSANT MEDICATIONS

DRUG	AUSTRALIA	NEW ZEALAND
Carbamazepine	Tegretol Teril Carbium Carbamazepine BC	Tegretol
Carbamazepine slow release	Tegretol CR	Tegretol CR
Clobazam	Frisium	Frisium
Clonazepam	Rivotril	Rivotril
Ethosuximide	Zarontin	Zarontin
Gabapentin	Neurontin Gantin	Neurontin
Lamotrigine	Lamictal	Lamictal
Levetiracetam	Keppra	
Nitrazepam	Mogadon Alodorm	Mogadon Insoma 5 Nitepam Nitraclos
Oxcarbazepine	Trileptal	Trileptal
Phenytoin/Phenytoin Sodium	Dilantin	Dilantin
Primidone	Mysoline	Mysoline
Sodium Valproate	Epilim Valpro	Epilim
Sulthiame	Ospolot	
Tiagabine	Gabitril	Gabitril
Topiramate	Topamax	Topamax
Vigabitrin	Sabril	Sabril

Appendix 3

Epilepsy Associations

EPILEPSY AUSTRALIA
The National Coalition of Australian Epilepsy Associations
National telephone: 1300 852 853
National website: epilepsyaustralia.com

Epilepsy Foundation of Victoria
818 Burke Rd
Camberwell VIC 3124
Telephone: 03 9805 9111
Email: epilepsy@epilepsy.asn.au
Website: www.epinet.org.au

Epilepsy Association ACT
27 Mulley St
Holder ACT 2611
Telephone: 02 6287 4555
Email: epilepsyact@bigpond.com

Epilepsy Association of Tasmania
250 Murray St
Hobart TAS 7000
Telephone: 03 6234 6967
Email: tasepilepsynw@easymail.com.au

Epilepsy Association of Western Australia
14 Bagot Rd
Subiaco WA 6008
Telephone: 08 9381 1187
Email: epilepsy@cygnus.uwa.edu.au

Epilepsy Association of South Australia
6 Woodville Rd
Woodville SA 5011
Telephone: 08 8445 6131
Email: easa@ozemail.com.au
Website: www.epicare.com.au/links/EASA_info.html

Epilepsy Queensland
411 Vulture St
Wooloongabba QLD 4102
Telephone: 07 3435 5000
Email: epilepsy@gil.com.au
Website: www.eqi.org.au

EPILEPSY ASSOCIATION
Suite 8, 44–46 Oxford St
Epping NSW 2121

GPO Box 9878 in your capital city
Telephone (Australia-wide) 1300 366 162
Email: epilepsy@epilepsy.org.au
Website: www.epilepsy.org.au

EPILEPSY NEW ZEALAND
610 Victoria St
Hamilton 2015
Telephone: 07 834 3556
Email: national@epilepsy.org.nz
Website: www.epilepsy.org.nz

References

Birch, C. *Regaining Compassion for Humanity and Nature*, University of NSW Press, Sydney, 1993.

Clark, M. *Puzzles of Childhood*, Penguin Books, Melbourne, 1989.

Mittan, R. 'Fear of Seizures' in Whitman, S. & Hermann, B. P. *Psychopathology in Epilepsy – Social Dimensions*, Oxford University Press, Oxford, 1986, pp. 90–121.

O'Donahue, N. V. *Epilepsies of Childhood*, Butterworth-Heinemann, London, 1985.

Scambler, G. *Epilepsy*, Routledge, London, 1989.

West, P. 'The Social Meaning of Epilepsy: Stigma as a Potential Explanation for Psychopathology in Children' in Whitman, S. & Hermann, B. P. *Psychopathology in Epilepsy – Social Dimensions*, Oxford University Press, Oxford, 1986, pp. 240–65.

Woodward, R. 'The Management of the Chronic Fatigue Syndrome' in *Me and You* Newsletter, September 1992.

Further Reading

Brown, R. *Young People and Epilepsy*, National Epilepsy Association of Australia, Sydney, 1993.

Chadwick, D. & Usiskin, S. *Living with Epilepsy*, Methuen, Melbourne, 1987.

Goss, S. *Ragged Owlet*, Houghton Mifflin Australia, Melbourne, 1989.

Laidlaw, M. V. & Laidlaw, J. *People with Epilepsy*, Churchill Livingstone, Edinburgh, 1984.

Sanders, L. & Thompson, P. *Epilepsy: A Practical Guide to Coping*, Crowood Press, London, 1989.

Scambler, G. *Epilepsy*, Routledge, London, 1989.

Schacter, S. C. *Brainstorms: Epilepsy in Our Words* (personal accounts of living with seizures), Raven Press, New York, 1993.

Shadows of Discrimination: A Study of Epilepsy in Queensland, Epilepsy Association of Queensland, Brisbane, 1993.

Whitman, S. & Hermann, B. P. *Psychopathology in Epilepsy – Social Dimensions*, Oxford University Press, Oxford, 1986.

Yanko, S. *Coming to Terms with Epilepsy*, Allen & Unwin, Sydney, 1993.

Index